Joseph Anthony Slota III & Erica Slota

CAN'T?
JUST
DID!

Win the Fight for Your Life
with Resilience, Faith, and Family

This book is dedicated to all of the medical professionals who cared for me and guided me to health, most important of whom are our amazing family and friends. We could not have gotten this far without each one of you.

FOREWORD

For years, I've watched patients go through courses of neurological rehabilitation with all levels of determination. Some people maintain a highly optimistic attitude, while others spend months in a state of depression with no motivation to recover. The majority of patients fall somewhere in between, but once in a while there's someone who stands out in a way that changes you as a practitioner.

From the moment I introduced myself to Joe and his father, I immediately knew he'd be someone who not only would succeed in his rehabilitation, but also would use his experience to make a difference in the world. Joe was the type of patient who met every challenge I threw at him with fierce determination, which in turn pushed me to be an even better physical therapist. On a group outing before his discharge, Joe was nervous and anxious, yet excited to walk and climb stairs within the community. As we stepped out the door, we discovered it was raining, which usually deters patients from attempting various outdoor activities. I challenged Joe to walk in the rain while carrying an umbrella over uneven pavement and up and down curbs. This was not an easy feat for someone who was still learning to walk safely, let alone walk while carrying a heavy object. Joe, of course, succeeded beyond my expectations; he was one of those rare cases that excelled every step of the way.

What Joe didn't realize was that while he thanked me profusely for the help and support I provided, I believe he had more of an impact on me than I had on him. His infectious smile, robust sense of humor, and unconditional persistence are what gave him the ability to achieve all of his goals. Those same qualities left a mark on each healthcare worker and fellow patient who had contact with Joe during his rehabilitation, including me. I consider it a privilege and an honor to have played a small role in Joe's recovery, and I look forward to the profound effect he will have on the world as people learn his story.

Jenna Tucker, PT, DPT, NCS, CBIS
Physical Therapist and Board Certified Neurological Specialist

I am a walking proof that anything is possible if you want it badly enough. What I thought was an average Sunday in June of 2013 turned into the last "normal" day I would spend in a long time.

PROLOGUE - WAKING UP

(JOE)

I FEEL LIKE I'm waking up after sleeping for days. It feels like something is holding my eyelids closed as I struggle to open them. I've felt groggy before, but never like this. When they do open, it's hard to see. I can't focus on much. Where am I? Who is here? Why the hell is a mitt strapped tightly over my right hand? Is this a joke? Am I boxing again? I can't speak. There's a tube coming out of my throat. I look down and can make out a loose—fitting, thin, hospital gown. Clearly, something is wrong with me. I can feel my heart beating strongly as anxiety takes me over. Where is my family? Am I okay?

I look over to my right, and I see my parents standing at my bedside, gazing down at me with serious, but comforting looks. Finally, I see people I recognize, people who always make me feel comfortable. I'm not in any pain at all, which is odd because I see so many tubes, machines, and wires. I must be on a ton of medication. I'm so confused. What is happening? I try to speak and can't. I'm petrified, but I want my family to know I love them. What can I do? Ah, my mitt! I lift my right arm, tap on my heart twice, and reach out to them, hoping that they'll understand my gesture. I want to let them know that I love them with all of my heart, and that I'm okay. I see tears pool in their eyes as they attempt to smile reassuringly. Everyone seems so scared and emotional. As I scan the room, I hear a nurse say to my parents in a calm tone, "Do you mind leaving for a bit? We will call you back in as soon as he's ready."

I'm still confused, and now I'm more anxious. Why are they asking them to leave? Why can't they stay? When will they be back? I follow them out of the room with my eyes, and then they're gone. What is going on? Inside, I begin to panic.

I hear the scraping of metal as a nurse pulls the curtain around my bed. I notice that I can't move my left side, at all, but I assume I'm just strapped in tight so I won't touch anything. Finally, a doctor walks up to me and leans over the bed, his face serious. He speaks with a heavy Eastern European accent. "Joseph, on the count of three, I want you to breathe out." Maybe he just wants to check my breathing. "One, two…" On his three count, I see stars as he pulls the breathing tube from my mouth. The discomfort shoots through my lips, tongue, and throat all at once. I wouldn't wish this feeling on my worst enemy! I spit up as the tube comes out. My mouth is so dry, and the tube has made a nasty bruise on my lips. I want to speak, but I can't.

Frustration mixed with discomfort and pain makes it difficult for me to stay calm. I wait a bit as I try to muster enough moisture in my mouth and throat to speak. I look over and see a nurse through blurry vision. In the best voice I can manage, I say to her, "Don't scare my mom. She's a very nice lady."

The nurse speaks to me in an exceedingly mellow tone. "Joe, my name is Dani. I'm your nurse. How are you feeling? Are you in any pain?"

"No, but my lips, throat, and tongue are really sore," I say, using all the moisture I have left in my mouth to answer her.

"Okay, that's normal. We'll give you something to take care of that."

Dani is moving briskly around the room, pushing buttons and checking my body. It's so hard for me to keep up with her. Everything is still blurry. As I watch Dani move around, I hear my sister, Erica, and my parents, their voices getting louder as they near the room. They're finally back! They'll help me understand why I'm here.

I look at them and the doctor. My parents and sister are the only three people I've seen in here without scrubs on. I must look confused, because I have no idea what's going on. "What happened to me?"

The doctor said, "Joe, you were born with an AVM, an arteriovenous malformation, in your brain, and it ruptured."

What is this guy talking about? What does that even mean? I feel stupid. I hear the words he is saying, but nothing registers. Nothing makes any sense. I look at my parents, puzzled. "What is happening to me?"

"Everything will be okay. We're not going anywhere," they say, and I know they are trying to keep me calm. The stress and concern in their eyes cannot be hidden.

"Joe!" I hear coming from four different voices in unison as I look to my left. My grandparents, my Zia (*aunt* in Italian), and Uncle Vinnie walk into the room. They seem calm and keep talking to me about how much they care for and love me. I can't tell if they're really calm or trying to hide their emotions. In the corner of my eye, I see Erica. She looks sad and frightened. I know that many people wouldn't know this about her, but I am so close to my sister that there is no way she can hide how she feels.

Okay, this is bad. I need to keep a smile on everyone's face, I say to myself.

And then, like a freight train tearing down the tracks, it hits me. I remember why I'm here.

JUNE 9TH (JOE AND ERICA)

(JOE)

MAN, WHAT A night! I thought as I slowly opened my eyes. I noticed a bit of pounding in my head, but it was nothing breakfast couldn't take care of. But, not yet, I thought. I lay in my king-size bed and stared at the ceiling. I was so happy I had finally got to go out. It had been a long time. I had been saving money for the last few months since I bought my townhouse. I'd given myself a great, much needed night out with my friends. We went to some local bars and got a chance to unwind and have some fun.

After lying in bed for an extra ten minutes, I went downstairs to make some breakfast. I decided I wanted whole wheat waffles with peanut butter and bananas. I'd have to stick to my diet; the night before had definitely been a cheat night.

My phone rang loudly, which did not help my headache. It was Anthony, one of my best friends since childhood.

"Hey man, what's up?" I said as I put the waffles in the toaster.

"I'm in the neighborhood taking a walk with Fiorella." That was his girlfriend, now his wife. "Can we stop by for a bit before I leave on my business trip?"

"Sure, come on by. I'm just making breakfast."

It was always fun to reminisce with my friends. We always had a good time together, so I looked forward to seeing them. After a half-hour conversation about the previous night, sharing some laughs, and talking about our plans for the next few weeks, they left. I glanced at the clock. I had plans to see my friend, Sarah. She was probably already on her way, so I figured I'd call her to check in.

"Hi, Sarah, how far away are you?" I asked when she answered, excited to show another friend my new house. I had purchased a two-bedroom townhouse in Morristown, New Jersey. I really enjoyed having friends and family over. I was extraordinarily proud of it.

"Hey, Joe. I'm about fifteen minutes away." Sarah sounded happy to hear me so excited. I couldn't help it. I'd worked hard to get where I was.

When Sarah arrived, we toured the downstairs portion of the house so she could see all the work I'd put into it, as well as my awesome TV with surround sound.

As I was guiding her upstairs, I felt a headache coming on. This headache was different from any I'd ever had before. It felt like brain freeze after eating ice cream too quickly, only I could also feel the iciness flowing through my veins, and I had the worst cramping in my head I'd ever felt in my life. The pain didn't subside even a little.

"Sarah, give me a second. I have such a bad headache. I'll be right back." I went into my master bathroom.

By then, I was getting cold sweats. Maybe it would help if I put pressure above my eyes. I held my head in my hands, pressing firmly. I waited a few seconds, but the pain only got worse. My arms and legs were starting to tingle as if they were falling asleep. The sweating was profuse. Beads of sweat dripped off my face and arms. I sat on the floor to see if the cool tile would provide some relief. Putting my phone next to me, I just lay there until I somehow found the strength to call my sister.

Each ring seemed to last an eternity. "Pick up, Erica, please," I whispered.

"Hey, Joe! What's up?" She was clearly excited to hear from me.

"Erica, I'm in so much pain. I have a really bad headache; I don't know what to do." I was panicking. "Where are you? I need help."

"You sound horrible, Joe! Did you take anything? Are you alone?"

"No, I feel like I'm going to pass out. My friend is downstairs."

"Hold on, Joe. I'm going to put Uncle Todd on the phone so he can tell you what to do." Our uncle is a doctor.

"What's wrong, Joe?" Uncle Todd said as he took the phone.

"I have a really bad headache above my eyes. I'm in so much pain."

"It sounds like you might have a cluster headache or maybe an atypical migraine. You can start by taking some acetaminophen and relaxing. See if it will subside. Let me know if it worsens or does not improve."

As we were about to say goodbye, I heard my sister ask for the phone back.

"Joe," she said, sounding nervous, "can you try to take the medicine?"

"I don't know if I can." It took nearly every ounce of energy I had left to answer her.

"Call 911, now. Tell your friend to leave the door open for them. I'm on my way," she said.

I dropped the phone as I started to vomit. Summoning up every bit of strength I had, I yelled, "Sarah, leave the door open and go. Please, I'm sorry." I felt like a horrible person, but the pain was so bad I just wanted her to go. I heard her pleading with me, but I just kept yelling, "Please go."

I picked up my phone, and dialed 911. "Help me," I said. "I have a really bad headache, and I'm vomiting. I don't want to die!"

"Sir, what's your address? I'll send someone over, now."

I gave her my address, and one last time, I cried to her, "Please hurry. I don't want to die."

I hung up and called Erica again.

"Joe, are you okay?" Erica asked as she answered. Her voice was shaky.

"No," I said, and then I dry-heaved over the toilet. I had nothing left in my system. I knew I needed help, and I needed it fast.

"Zia and I are on our way. Don't hang up. Is your friend still there?

"I don't know," I answered, not remembering that I asked her to leave. "Sarah!" I yelled. No response.

"Joe, give me your garage code so Zia can call 911 and let them know in case they can't get in."

I gave Erica my code, and could hear Zia in the background, trying to get in touch with the 911 operator.

"Sir, EMTs! Can we come in?" a man's voice yelled.

"Please hurry. I don't want to die," I answered, unable to get up.

"Sir, your leg is blocking the door. Can you move it?" a female voice called.

"If I could move my leg, I'd be in your truck by now," I responded, sounding like a smart ass but not meaning to be one.

Finally, a hand reached around the door and grabbed my leg by the pants. They were able to slide me over enough to open the door. The EMTs rushed in and put an oxygen mask on me. They told me to take a few deep breaths and that I was going to be okay.

I was scared. I couldn't understand what was happening to me. I just wanted the pain to go away.

"Sir, we're going to put you in a chair and get you downstairs into the ambulance. If you have any energy left at all, we need you to help lift yourself up."

I had no energy left at all. My vision was becoming blurry as I felt an oxygen mask being placed on my face.

"Sir, try to relax. We're going to get you out of here." I wasn't convinced.

"Joe, Zia is here. Don't worry. You're not alone," I heard my aunt call from my bedroom. As the paramedics were opening an accordion chair to help me get downstairs, my aunt said, her voice trembling a little, "Joe, I love you, but I have to ask: Did you do anything you weren't supposed to last night? Any drugs, or maybe hanging out with people who might have put something in your drink?"

In hindsight, I knew that she knew better, but everyone must have been confused as to what was happening to me. It was becoming more difficult to speak. I shook my head no. At this point, I could make out four EMT workers in my bathroom. They finally got me into the chair, and then my eyes closed. Everything seemed to happen in chunks with some spaces that I don't remember.

"Joe, I'm here, and I won't let anything happen to you, do you understand me? I'm not going anywhere. I love you. Nod if you can hear me," Erica said, sounding worried but honest. I nodded, but I still couldn't open my eyes. They felt sealed shut.

"We're going to take you for a CAT scan now, Joe." This voice also had a nervous quality, but it was unrecognizable. How could they take me for a CAT scan in my bathroom? I was extremely confused.

That was the last voice I would hear before the most difficult experience of my life.

(ERICA)

"THIS LOOKS AWESOME!" I said to my grandmother, looking at the plate of homemade ravioli in front of me. Who could pass up her cooking?

I had gone to my aunt's house to have a late lunch with family. My parents were down the shore for the day, and I had talked to Joe earlier in the morning to see if he wanted to join us. Since we both had moved, I felt like we hadn't seen each other as often as usual. He told me a friend was coming over to see his new house, so he didn't think he could make it. I was disappointed, but I completely understood.

On my third ravioli, I made a mess. "Yeah, I need like fifteen napkins when I eat," I joked as I got up to get more napkins. As I did,

I stopped in my tracks. My phone ringer was never on, but at that moment, I had an odd feeling that I should check my phone. I turned back around to where it was lying on the table, and there on the screen was an old picture of Joe and me on St. Patrick's Day—and now he was calling. Odd that I'd checked my phone at that very moment.

"Hey, Joe. Did you change your mind?" I asked, excited at the thought of seeing him. We had both moved into new homes in February, so I hadn't seen my brother as frequently as I once did. We've always had such a close-knit relationship. Some people say that they are best friends with a sibling, but when we say it, we mean it.

When Joe told me about his headache, I knew I had to get moving. I grabbed my phone and my purse and ran from the air conditioned house into the summer heat. It hit me like a wall of bricks, just like hearing Joe's voice on the phone. As I started my car, I plugged Joe's address into my navigator. I was trying not to let my nerves get to me, but I couldn't help but fumble with the buttons. I heard my aunt yelling at me to open the door so she could come with me. She jumped in, and I sped off in the direction that my navigation indicated. I hoped I was going the quickest way to his house. I worried that I might get lost, which was a regular occurrence for me. I have no sense of direction whatsoever. I wondered if they might take him to the hospital before I got there and what I should do. I had to think.

My phone rang. I saw Joe's name on the screen and answered, frantic.

"Erica, I don't know what to do. I'm scared," Joe mumbled into the phone. He sounded muffled by something.

My stomach was in a complete knot. "Joe it's okay. We're coming. Nothing is going to happen to you. Just try to stay awake and try to open the door so the paramedics can come in. I love you. Just hang in there," I shouted into my Bluetooth. I had no idea if what I said was true, but he needed the encouragement at that moment.

My aunt and I continued to talk to Joe, hoping to make sure that everything was being taken care of. Hearing his voice decline by the second is something I know that my aunt and I will never forget. He was mumbling, and less and less intelligible. Then, he stopped responding in words we could comprehend. Joe was in the bathroom, immobile, and I was concerned that the paramedics wouldn't be able to get into his house. I asked my aunt to call 911 to make sure they had Joe's garage code in case the door was locked. Once we knew the paramedics had arrived, we were relieved to know that Joe was no longer alone.

"I'm Joe's sister," I told them. I'm on my way there right now. He has me on speaker phone." I hoped that they would be able to give me an update on his condition.

"Ma'am, we have to go," they said, hanging up Joe's phone.

Rage flooded me. "What the hell is their problem? He's there in pain and they just hang up on me?" I shouted.

"Erica, it's a liability to have someone listen in," my aunt said.

"Crap! I took the wrong freakin' exit!" I yelled, frustrated with myself for getting lost once again. Even though my navigation was on, I had too many emotions going through my body to be able to focus on the annoying generic voice of my GPS.

"Relax, we can't help him if we don't get there in one piece," my aunt said. I could tell she was nervous, but trying to hold it together for my benefit.

As we pulled in front of his house, I could see the ambulance and the EMT truck.

"Zia, I'll drop you off in front of his house and then I'll go park the car. I don't want him to feel like he's alone."

"Okay, I'll see you inside," she replied.

I found a spot in the lot near his house. I looked at the ambulance, and then at the rosary beads hanging from my windshield. "Lord, please let him be okay," I prayed, not knowing what I was about to see.

I ran inside the house as quickly as I could. I could hear voices upstairs. When I was halfway up the stairs, one of the workers said, "Ma'am, we're trying to get him down."

"Why can't he walk down?" I asked, confused.

Nobody answered me.

About two minutes later, I saw them carrying my brother down in a chair. It seemed to be happening in slow motion. Joe is not a small guy; it took a few of them to help him down the steps. They were slow and steady, which was really the only way to get him down without him falling or hurting himself.

The second I looked at my brother, I knew this wasn't going to be good. Beads of sweat dripped from his body. His left leg was hanging off the chair, his head was tilted to the left, and he was completely out of it. I wasn't expecting him to look like that. He looked like someone about to die. I felt as if I'd been punched in the stomach and nothing could help me breathe again.

"Joe, it's Erica. I'm right here, bud. I don't want you to worry. Everything is going to be okay," I said.

With my parents down the shore, I knew that I needed to make sure everything was handled the right way. What did I need to do? I had to think.

"Joe, where is your wallet? I need to get your insurance card. I also need your phone," I said, hoping he would be able to answer me. He grunted a bit but couldn't answer clearly. He pointed with his right hand, indicating the living room. I got his wallet, and just then, his phone rang as the paramedics were bringing it down from the bathroom. *Sarah* showed up in big letters. That was the girl who was there earlier. Maybe she knew what was wrong. Maybe she had done this to him! Wait—why was she gone? Where the hell *was* that girl? I knew it wasn't right for me to assume, but at that moment, I had nothing else to go with. I wanted answers.

Every thought known to man traveled through my head. When I answered Sarah's call, I bombarded the poor girl with a million questions. She seemed innocent enough, although I'm sure I came across as a lunatic. At that moment, nothing mattered but Joe. As the paramedics took Joe outside, it took everyone, including my aunt and me, to hold the gurney down so they could put Joe on it. Once they had secured him, the paramedics wheeled him toward the ambulance.

I had noticed one of the female workers staring at me throughout this ordeal. She had paid close attention to all that I did to try to help. As they were about to pull away, she looked at me again and yelled, "Hey, you're a good sister! Remember that." She is one of the few faces from that afternoon that I can still remember today.

"Zia, you go with him in the ambulance, and I'll drive my car to the hospital," I said.

I was dreading the call I needed to make to my parents. I braced myself.

"Hey, sweetheart! Nice to hear from you," my dad said when he answered.

"Dad, something is wrong with Joe. I don't want to scare you guys, but he doesn't look good. I made him call an ambulance. I think you guys should come home. They're taking him to the hospital."

My parents started packing up while asking me a million questions. I told them I would call them back once we had some answers. I didn't want them to drive frantically, so I kept my composure. The three most important people in my life were emotionally unavailable, and I felt completely alone.

The ride to the hospital was a complete blur. I drove, paying no mind to any of the cars around me. I had to get to there quickly. I was so overwhelmed with emotions that I didn't know how to handle myself. When I pulled into the hospital, I called my cousin Jenna. I updated her on what was going on, and she did her best to calm me down. I don't remember much of what I said, but I'm sure it probably sounded angry and didn't make much sense. I said goodbye and ran into the hospital to find Joe. I had to ask directions from about four different people. Each time, I could only half-listen and got lost. Once I finally found Joe, I felt much better. He was in a safe place where they would give him medicine and send him back home with us.

Joe was still out of it, so I kept reminding him that I was there and that he didn't have to worry. "I'm not going anywhere. I love you," I repeated over and again. I wouldn't let go of his hand. We had three people in scrubs in the room. I couldn't tell the doctors from the nurses.

And then it happened. It is still vivid in my memory as if it had happened yesterday. A doctor asked Joe to squeeze his hands. His right hand was fine, but he couldn't squeeze with his left.

"Joe, just try! I know you're tired, but please, show him that you can do it," I cried, begging him to snap out of it. I just couldn't understand why he wasn't listening or responding.

The doctor looked at me and then moved down to Joe's feet. He took his keys out of his pocket and slid the tip of his key along Joe's right foot. It flew up; clearly, his reflexes were working properly. He did the same on Joe's left foot, and nothing happened. A glance at my aunt's face, and I knew something was wrong. She blinked, but this time kept her eyes closed longer than she naturally would.

"Stop!" I yelled to the doctor. "Do it again! You didn't push hard enough!"

He ignored me, shouting to the other doctors and nurses in the room. "He needs a CAT scan, now!"

In seconds, the crowded room emptied. My uncle had shown up at some point during the craziness. He looked just as frightened as my aunt.

"What is happening? Tell me, now. He needs to be okay! He's my brother, he's my best friend, and I can't live without him. Is he going to live?" I repeated. Nobody could answer me, even though I was begging for reassurance with every fiber of my being. I couldn't breathe. I felt like someone was trying to suffocate me and there was nothing I could do to make it stop.

"We believe he had a stroke," the doctor said.

"He's twenty-six! That's impossible!" I yelled. "You have to save him! Save my brother. I love him; he's my best friend. Save my brother!" I kept yelling.

I don't know how loud I was yelling, and I didn't care. At that moment, the man who delivered this news became my enemy. Although I knew it was irrational, all I wanted was to make him stop speaking. I completely shut down. I could see the man speaking to my aunt and uncle, but I couldn't hear a word he was saying. Once he left, I looked at my family. They were clearly distraught but trying to keep it together for my sake. I cried to them, "I need him. I can't live without him. Zia, you and Mom are best friends. You can't live without her, just like I can't live without Joe. Someone needs to save him!"

My aunt told me to calm down and asked me to sit outside the room in the hallway. I knew she wanted to talk about the seriousness of the matter with my uncle, and although I would normally fight to be included in such a conversation, I didn't want to hear it. I just wanted someone to fix this. I found a seat and cried. I knew I had to call my parents. I dreaded making the phone call.

"Erica, how's Joe?" my dad asked. He was on the Bluetooth in the car, driving up from the shore with my mom. He sounded like he wanted to be calm for the sake of my mom, but it was obvious he was shook up.

"Joe, slow down!" I heard my mom yell in the background.

I knew I couldn't tell them all I knew about Joe's condition thus far. It was too dangerous for them to have to drive, knowing that their son was not doing well. But they did need to know it was serious.

"Dad, you guys need to drive safely. He...he doesn't look good. Just get here, okay?" I didn't know what to say. I always knew how to handle situations with my family. But this time, I was at a loss. I couldn't process what was happening myself, therefore I couldn't find the words to comfort anyone else.

"Did he vomit?" my mom asked.

I could tell by her voice that she was hoping for a certain response that I couldn't give her.

"Yes," I answered, wondering why she had asked.

"Oh my God, it's a stroke!" she screamed.

I couldn't understand how she knew, but I sensed that I should not confirm what she had said. The intensity of her scream told me that this was even worse than I had anticipated. I didn't know if I had said too much, but there was nothing more I could do.

"Just get here, guys. We'll be in the emergency room waiting room." I wanted my parents to be there so they could make this all go away. They had to make this better. Or at least come and tell me that it was a horrible dream.

I sat in that room and waited. My aunt and uncle sat on one side of the room, but I wanted to be alone. I needed to be.

Eventually, a man came in. I was hoping he would tell me that everything was okay and we could leave. But that wasn't the case. Instead, he told me that since I was Joe's sister, I needed to read some paperwork and sign it. The paperwork included information regarding Joe's wishes if something terrible should happen to him. This was the complete opposite of what I had hoped for. No sibling should ever have to process something like that. I stopped reading after the words "in case of death" came up on the paper. I cried, told him to just tell me where to sign, and I signed the paper.

I'm not sure how much time had passed, but a little bit later, my parents came in. I felt a sense of relief at first—until I realized that they were just as worried as I was. They stood there, scared out of their minds, crying. I hugged them as hard as I could. I could feel them both shaking, just as I had been ever since we received the news.

I wanted to talk to my brother, my voice of reason. When anything bad happened, he was the person I talked to. I felt so alone. Who was I supposed to go through this with? Not having him to talk to would be bad. Knowing that, potentially, I might never have him to talk to again was unbearable. In my twenty-eight years on the planet, I had never felt as lonely and sad. I would have endured any amount of physical pain to make my emotional pain subside.

OVERLOOK MEDICAL CENTER, MY HOME AWAY FROM HOME (JOE AND ERICA)

(JOE)

"ALL RIGHT, EVERYONE. Time for Joe to rest," I heard Dani say authoritatively. "Immediate family can stay for a bit, but everyone else needs to go. Sorry!"

Surprisingly, though, my extended family said goodbye and went back to the waiting room. It wasn't like them to leave a family member in need just because someone told them to. But this time, they listened. I'd later learn that the waiting room at Overlook Medical Center in Summit, New Jersey was a setting they had come to know all too well while they sat in fear of the outcome of my surgeries. It had become their home away from home. It was a place I'm sure they'd never want to see again.

I felt the need to make everyone laugh while my room was full of family and fake smiles. I could tell everyone had been nervous, so I made it my goal to lighten the mood and show them that I was fine. Now that it was just my parents and Erica in the room, I was able to take it all in. I looked at all the tubes connected to my body and listened to the consistent beeping of the annoying machines next to me. Then, I saw this clear, grenade-shaped container to my right. As I reached for it, I watched as each member of my family and the nurse all jumped, as if I were a toddler about to descend a staircase for the first time.

"No! Don't touch that!" my dad yelled. I stopped in my tracks.

"Okay. Well, what is it?" I asked, still frightened by everyone's response.

"It's a drain for excess fluid in your brain," Dani said nonchalantly, as if she had delivered this news to patients often.

I tried not to look worried, but now it hit me that I really had just undergone major brain surgery.

"You mean to tell me this is my brain juice next to me?"

The tension in the room finally released as everyone laughed. I'd later learn that these moments were very important to my family. They were scared that I would be in a bad place emotionally, so each time I laughed or made them laugh, it helped to give them hope that things could be okay.

"Listen, I'm a creative guy, and if you guys come out with some good ideas, I'll know where to find you. I know what you guys could do with someone's brain juice. Don't steal any of my ideas!" I laughed, trying my best to hide my concern for the situation.

Everyone had looked so tired that it was a relief to finally see them smile. I needed to understand what the situation was, though. I was there in that bed, hooked up to machines, and I had a grenade coming out of my head! Was I okay? What was happening? It seemed like they could tell that I was confused. That was when they began to explain to me in detail what I had gone through in the past 24 hours.

The surgery was an emergency due to a ruptured AVM, which, they explained, was a malformed area in which the high blood flow arteries meet the low blood flow veins. In my situation, the AVM was in my brain. This typically occurs a couple of weeks after conception and can be classified as a birth defect. I had gone through my entire life up to then without ever knowing that I had a ticking time bomb in my head. The first surgery, and the swiftness of the events leading up to it, had saved my life. If it hadn't been for Erica's intuition to tell me to call 911, the speed at which I arrived at the hospital, the prayers and support of my family in the waiting room, and the amazing doctors and nurses who were on call that night, I would not be here today.

The first surgery was a success. The bleeding from the ruptured AVM had caused pressure to build in my head. The emergency craniotomy surgery removed a portion of my skull, which relieved the pressure on my brain. If it hadn't been done when it was, my situation could have been much worse.

I was so tired…

(ERICA)

"THANK GOD," I whispered to my parents as Joe slept. I knew he was on a ton of pain medication and needed his rest. Normally, we would all have left the room and let him rest, but that day we felt such relief that we selfishly needed to sit by Joe's side, just to watch him breathe. I stared at his chest. I thought about the papers I had signed and the conversations we'd had with doctors in the 24 hours that we'd been in the hospital. I couldn't believe that this was real. Little things started to bother me. The smell of antibacterial soap still makes me sick to this day. No matter where I went during that time, I couldn't escape that smell. Soon, it became a trigger for my anxiety.

"I think he's going to be okay," my dad whispered to my mom. Both had tears in their eyes. "He looks and sounds much better than I imagined. We need to be strong and have faith. No crying in front of him, okay?" he said, looking at both of us.

With tears streaming down our faces, my mom and I nodded our heads in agreement.

The night before, the doctor had come into the waiting room to talk to the family after Joe's surgery. I remember watching him walk into the room. His scrubs were on, he seemed tired, but most of all, he seemed concerned. I was right. His words cut like a knife. He explained where the bleed was and told us that he couldn't be sure how Joe would be when he woke up. When we asked him to clarify, he said, "The area of the bleed could have a harmful effect on his vision. We stopped the bleed early, but we can't be sure that Joe will be able to walk again. It all depends on how he is when he wakes up. There's nothing more that you guys can do here tonight. You need to go home and get some sleep. Come back in the morning."

His words hit me like a freight train. Why was this happening to Joe? He didn't deserve this. He hadn't done anything wrong. I felt like the blood had been drained from my body, and I was just a walking corpse.

Before the doctor left, my mom said to him, "Take care of my boy." This became a regular occurrence. She said those words to every medical professional we encountered.

Being in the room with Joe the next day, knowing that he was able to see us and talk with us, was a huge relief. Our Joe had survived. The Slota family has four pieces. With one of those pieces missing, we would never have been whole again. Now, we didn't have to worry about that.

My brother and I have always known how much our parents love us. They've been vocal about their feelings and made it a point to put us first, no matter what. They raised us to love each other as siblings and best friends. Watching my parents in the ER waiting room was absolute hell. I was worried about my brother, but I was also worried about them. I remember how they had stormed through the waiting room door, both with tears streaming down their faces, hoping that one of us would tell them that everything was fine. But we couldn't. They ran over to me. The three of us huddled together and cried. I knew my parents were dependable, but from that day forward, their love, determination, and strength could never be matched by any other parents on this planet.

While we waited in Joe's room and watched him sleep, my dad talked to the nurses and learned whatever he could about the machines

Joe was hooked up to. He made sure the room was kept at a comfortable temperature and that the nurses looked Joe over every time they set foot in Room 518. He built a rapport with every individual that was associated with the care of my brother.

"Do you really think he's going to be okay?" I whispered, finally able to speak. I hadn't said much during the past 24 hours. The thought of possibly losing my brother was still too much to think about. I didn't know how to verbalize what I was thinking because I couldn't process any of what had happened.

"Yes, We need to be strong. You heard him. He's cracking jokes! Don't let him see you upset," my dad said, trying to be strong for us. I could tell he was nervous and unsure, but he wouldn't entertain the idea of Joe not being okay.

"We all need to say a prayer. Let's go to the chapel again and let him sleep," Mom suggested.

Although we wanted to stay with Joe, Dad and I knew she was right; he needed his rest. We each kissed Joe's hand, careful not to wake him. We walked to the chapel. The dark room was one that we knew well, since we had taken turns sitting in there the night before. Each of us wrote notes in the book begging God to look down and protect Joe. This time, I kneeled and I thanked God for keeping him alive. Each time I pray, I ask God to look over each member of my family as I list them in my mind, one by one. This time, I asked God to give me a sign that Joe was going to be okay.

Please, God, anything at all, I prayed. I just need to know that Joe will be okay.

I opened my eyes and then the lights flickered. My mouth dropped open. I knew instantly it was the sign I had been looking for. Mom noted my expression and gave me a look, her eyes asking me what was wrong. I stared into her bloodshot eyes and said, "That was my sign that Joe is going to be okay."

We both smiled despite our tears and hugged each other tight.

JUNE 11TH – REQUEST FOR PRAYER

(JOE)

"DAD, DO YOU think Father Martin can come to visit me?" I asked my father in a raspy, quiet tone. I was still groggy from all of my pain medication.

"Sure, I can call and ask him to come by this week," my dad replied, smiling. He was already in my room at six a.m. so I wouldn't wake up alone.

I've always had a strong faith, even though I was never a consistent churchgoer. Father Martin had been the priest in my family's church for many years. I had a lot of respect for him because he always had a special way with his words. He was comforting and warm, and his Irish accent was calming and always made me feel comfortable. He gave my Grandpa Joe his last rites, and I wanted to see him so he could say a special prayer with me.

When Dad returned from making the call, he said, "Okay, Joe. Father Martin told me that he would look at his schedule and try to be here by the end of the week."

"Perfect! Thanks so much." I had never needed God more than I did then.

As the day progressed, I had more family visitors. My grandparents came by with my Uncle Vinnie. My cousins were there by my side, too.

I was talking to my sister when I heard my dad say excitedly, "Joe, you have a visitor."

Being the smart ass I was during my stay at the hospital, I quipped, "Is it a hot blonde?"

Everyone was silent until my sister, giving me a look, said with a smirk, "Not quite."

All of a sudden, I heard that soothing Irish voice I remembered from throughout my childhood say, "Joseph, how are you feeling?"

Wow, he had gotten there quickly. I couldn't believe in just a few hours he had made the trip over to see me. Great! I really had just called my priest a hot blonde. Oh, boy!

"Well, I was way off, wasn't I?" I joked, causing everyone in the room to erupt in laughter.

I had gotten myself out of that one.

Father Martin looked at me for a moment and then whispered in my ear, "Joseph, I came here to pray for you to get well. How are you feeling?"

I nodded to Father Martin. "I'm okay, but I feel horrible that I haven't been a good enough Catholic."

"Joseph, we can't all be perfect all the time, but it's important that you ask God for forgiveness. You're a good man, and God forgives our sins," he replied, proving to me once again that his words, unlike the words of anyone else, could bring calm over me.

Together, everyone in the room began to pray the Our Father. I started to cry as comfort washed over me. In that moment, I felt my grandfather was with us. He had passed away six years earlier. The feeling was surreal. I couldn't see him, but I felt he was there.

"He is here with us! He's here! I know he's in the room with us," I cried out to my family.

"Who is here?" Erica asked, concerned.

"He's here with us right now!" I said again, not realizing that everyone was waiting for answers.

"Joe, who is here?" Erica asked again. This time she was touching my leg as if to protect me.

"Grandpa Joe. He's in the room with us now. I can feel him. He's here," I said frantically.

Everyone in the room had tears streaming down their faces. We all looked to Father Martin for some clarity as to what was going on. Father Martin nodded as if it wasn't the first time he had seen something like this. A feeling that I was being comforted came over me. I felt my grandfather sent me the message that he would protect me throughout this battle.

I didn't yet know how important a part faith would play in my recovery, but that was when I knew that everything was going to be just fine.

REFLECTION

(JOE)

ALTHOUGH FRIENDS AND family surrounded me throughout my hospital stay, I had time alone that I spent reflecting on my childhood.

I spent my early childhood years in Lake Hiawatha, New Jersey, with my sister, Erica, my father, Joe, and my mother, Maria. Although we're two years apart, Erica and I have always been best friends. I always wanted to do everything Erica did, even if I was too young. Erica was always the first to convince our parents to allow me to do the same things. We spent most of our time after school outside, playing sports with the kids in the neighborhood. Unlike many other parents, our parents were always around to make Erica and me happy. We took many vacations together, even if only to one of our favorite spots in Lancaster, Pennsylvania. Although it wasn't like a trip to a sunny beach, we loved being together and found the life of the Amish interesting. The ride there was a long one, so our parents would give each of us a box of sports cards to occupy us. Sports cards have been a hobby for both of us ever since, and that now includes memorabilia collecting. While in Lancaster, Mom loved to shop at the outlet stores. My father wasn't the biggest fan of shopping, and of course, neither were Erica and I, being kids. The three of us always found a way to have fun. Typically, we'd go to an empty area of the parking lot to play a game of catch and invent our own games.

We lived around the corner from my maternal grandparents, Rosa and Joe, and my Uncle Vinnie. This was a second home for Erica and me. We would run in between the houses to my grandparents' house to play soccer with Grandpa, cook with Grandma, or simply enjoy the food she cooked for us. Vinnie was always up for taking Erica and me to Volunteer's Park to play basketball or catch. On some weekends, Erica and I slept over at our grandparents' house, and Vinnie would take us to the local video store to rent wrestling matches that we'd watch until we fell asleep. In the morning, we'd continue watching while Grandma made us breakfast. And while eating breakfast, it was not uncommon to watch soccer with Grandpa on Italian television. Many Sunday mornings rang with screams of "Goal!" from the television, followed by a lot of fast-talking Italian.

Every other Sunday, my paternal grandpa (also Joe), came to visit us from Jersey City. Erica and I always knew when he had arrived because we could smell the mixture of cigar from his clothing and fresh pastries from a great bakery in Jersey City. It was always fun to see him, hear stories about our father when he was growing up, and listen to them trade jokes. Typically, it concluded with my grandfather looking at my dad and saying, "Oh, Docky (his nickname for my father), don't be such a goddamn jackass!" And then both of them would laugh. As you can see, weekends were always eventful and full of laughs.

My mother's sister Rossana, who we called Zia (*Aunt* in Italian), also played a big part in Erica's and my childhood. She did not live around the corner from us but would often come to visit and take us to the movies or to where she lived for sleepovers. Zia was very much a second mother to us. We went to her for advice just as we did with our own mom, and we never felt nervous about asking. Erica and I loved to hang out with Zia, especially when she let us do things we were normally not allowed to do at home, like play hockey on her hardwood floors with a broom and a ball.

Just when I thought my family life couldn't get any better, Zia and Uncle (Todd) told us they were expecting. Nine months later, our cousin Jenna was brought into the world, followed by Luke four years later. They were like siblings to Erica and me. I promised Zia I would always be there to help and watch over them, no matter what, especially given that there was more than an eight-year age gap between us.

My family has always been there for me through the difficulties in my life, and I for them. It is understood that we can call on each other for assistance whenever it's needed, with no questions asked. For my whole life, I have tried to be there for every one of my family members, wanting to be the strong one. Never in my life did I think I would be in a situation where all my family members would rally on June 9, 2013, to get me through the biggest struggle of my life. That day has forever changed my life.

HERE WE GO: SURGERY TWO (JOE AND ERICA)

(JOE)

I WAS CONFIDENT, optimistic, and excited to get it over with. At the same time, I was nervous as hell, but I couldn't show my family. They had been through enough worry. I didn't really know what the surgery was about, but one day, I knew it would all make sense. I needed to put my faith in God and trust that my family and the doctors were doing what was best for me.

Every time someone walked into my room, my heart skipped a beat. "Is it time?" I asked my dad.

"Soon, Joe. Hang in there," he said, clearly hearing anxiety in my voice.

Erica and Mom kept coming in and out of the room. I didn't know it then, but I know now that they were taking breaks because they were so worried. They didn't want me to see them cry, so they would leave when they felt that they were going to get emotional. Later, I'd find out that that day's surgery was extremely important. The first surgery had been emergency surgery; they had removed a portion of my skull to alleviate the pressure on my brain caused by the bleed. The second surgery was a "gluing" process to keep the AVM from bleeding further.

Surgery was scheduled for nine a.m., but an unexpected emergency surgery had delayed it. The minutes felt like hours. I kept thinking about the person going through the emergency surgery. I couldn't believe I, too, had gone through it and wasn't aware of it. My family must have been so scared. Had time dragged on for them, as well? I decided to take a nap so the time would go by more quickly.

"Okay, Joe, we're ready," I heard, just as I was about to fall into a deep sleep. I opened my eyes quickly and felt my heart frantically beating.

"What time is it?" I asked.

"Three p.m. Sorry for the delay. Sometimes the emergency surgeries come out of nowhere and we have to get them done."

"No worries," I said, distracted by the thought of having to be the next to go.

I looked over at my family and saw their horrible acting. They were trying to be as strong as could be. I couldn't imagine then and I can't imagine now how hard it must have been for them to see me get wheeled away each time.

"I got this," I said to my family, reassuring them and reassuring myself. "Let's get the show on the road."

(ERICA)

THE WALLS FELT like they were closing in. It was hard to breathe. When I saw Joe being wheeled away, he looked happy. Was he for real, I wondered, or was he doing it for us? Seeing him being taken away brought back memories from the day before. I had watched Joe get wheeled away from his house and get driven away by an ambulance, and now this. Each time, I worried that he'd be wheeled away and I would never see him again.

As soon as Joe was out of our line of vision, we decided to walk to the chapel as a family. I watched as my mom signed the book in the front. She looked calm, but I knew her better than that. My mom has such class. Even in the most difficult of times, she stands out among others. The way she signed the book, the way she took her seat, even the way she prayed—she did it all to perfection. I hoped that God was listening to her prayer, because Joe needed to be okay. I couldn't be without him, and I couldn't be the only child that my parents watched grow up. Suddenly, I felt more pressure, and my already wet eyes filled up even more.

I took the pen to write my note to God. "Dear God, please watch over my brother while he's in surgery. Please help him and all of the other people suffering in the hospital," I wrote, feeling hopeful, awkward, and yet relieved to get my thoughts on paper.

I went to my seat, and then knelt down to say a prayer. I asked God to look over every member of my family. I mentioned them all silently by name. This time, I could see I was haggling with God: "God, please make sure Joe is okay. I know you have my Grandpa Joe up there with you. Please help my brother through. He's a good boy, and I can't live my life without him here. I'll do anything. Please, just make sure he's okay."

Once I was finished praying, I lifted my eyes and saw my mom. She was looking at me almost as if she had heard every word of my prayer. I was happy to have my family with me, but at the same time I wished I could shake them, make them open up to me. Mom wouldn't eat. She wouldn't break down and cry with me. She seemed so deep in thought that she couldn't let any words out. I wanted to get through to her and make her talk to me. Dad was just as worried about her, I could tell. There was nothing anyone could do or say to relieve our worries. Our fate was in God's hands. My extended family was there, as well. As close as we had always been, a silence took over now. Nobody could find the right words to say. We all hurt to our core because one of our teammates was down. And there was nothing any of us could do to change that.

Later, when Dr. C came into the waiting room, I tried my best to read his face. It seemed I had been waiting an eternity to see him walk in with his scrubs on. I could hardly wait for the words to come out of his mouth. I needed to know how Joe was. The doctor looked tired. Or was he worried? What if he was about to deliver bad news?"

"All good," he said. "I think we got it all," he said.

It felt like someone had rewired my heart and plugged it back in. "So, he's okay? He's going to be better, now?" I cried, cutting him off unintentionally but needing to know.

"We got the AVM glued to stop the bleeding. Now, we have to see how he does," Dr. C replied.

I could tell he was trying to sound as positive as possible without giving us false hope. I wasn't good with anticipation. I had never felt so much anxiety before. Having to wait for results that could potentially be life-altering was horrific.

I tried to listen as he continued his report, but I couldn't. Joe was okay. That was all I knew. I don't know how I mustered the strength to wait for these updates from doctors. To this day, I can't figure out how I was able to sit in a chair and keep myself from falling apart while my brother was in surgery. I guess faith is a unique phenomenon. I sometimes feel that God took hold of my hand and wouldn't let go. Somehow, He kept my family in His arms and guided us. I know this sounds clichéd, but I really have no other explanation for the time we spent in limbo. I'm an anxious person by nature. Throughout my life, I've questioned many things. For some reason, although this was the toughest, most horrific time of my life, I questioned absolutely nothing. God was either going to guide us toward my brother's recovery or leave us in the dust. I am so thankful that the latter option was not in His plans.

TWENTY-SEVENTH BIRTHDAY

(JOE)

"DO YOU THINK the nurses are going to get mad?" I heard my sister ask my parents.

"No. It's his birthday. If they need space, we'll move everything. You worry too much," my dad said, reassuring my sister.

"He's up! Happy birthday!" my family shouted in unison. The noise was piercing. As I opened my eyes, everything was a bit blurry. I saw balloons, cards, and gifts everywhere. I definitely had not planned to spend my birthday in a hospital, that's for sure.

"Thanks, guys," I replied, still groggy from the previous day's surgery. I loved my family. I had no other words to explain how much I appreciated them. They didn't even think of not celebrating my birthday.

"Joe, we love you so much. You are truly a gift to us. Twenty-seven years ago, you were born, and we received the best gift in the whole world," my dad said with a tear in his eye.

"Well, what the hell!" my sister said, killing the sappy moment with a joke. "I guess the gift you received twenty-eight years ago wasn't all that great."

For the first time in a few days, we laughed together as a family. Looking back, I've definitely realized that when you have a good core foundation as a family, you truly can get through anything.

Mom said, "I have the best family in the world. Thank God. We all need to say a prayer today that we're able to be here. All four of us are here together, and that's because of our faith. We need to say a prayer."

Today, my mom finally had some color. She still looked worried, of course, but more positive and like herself.

Two weeks before, I had been planning to have a "beer Olympics" at my new place to celebrate with my friends. When that day came, I was fighting for my life. Of all the gifts in the room, the best gift was being with my family.

"Joe! Happy birthday!" I heard a bunch of familiar voices shout. I cautiously lifted my head to confirm who was talking to me.

In walked the rest of my extended family with even more gifts. I wondered whether there were any rules about the number of people allowed in the ICU. There probably were, but my family wouldn't be the ones to obey that rule. I actually felt a bit sad for the patients in the other rooms. Not many people were going in to visit. Sometimes when it was quiet, I'd listen for voices from their rooms. I had yet to hear anyone.

"I have a bunch of cards here from all of us and your friends. Do you want me to read some of them to you?" Erica asked me, purposely steering me away from my deep thoughts. We are so close that she seems to know when I'm sad before anyone else.

"Sure, that sounds good," I said, even though I was extremely exhausted and drowsy. I can't remember everything that was written in those cards. What I do remember is the feeling I had after listening to them. Lots of my friends and family had gone out of their way to make me happy. I couldn't have asked for better people in my life. For a guy who had gone through major trauma and surgery and was in a lot of pain, I was more than content to know how much people cared about me. The feeling left me overwhelmed with emotion.

Later that evening, my family left. The doctors advised them to go so that I could get some rest. I could tell that they felt guilty leaving, but I assured them that I would be okay. And I could call if I needed them. Unfortunately for them, I couldn't really make out the time on the clock. I called at random hours, not realizing how late it was.

"What's wrong?" My mom would say when she answered the phone.

"I love you. I just wanted to tell you," I'd reply to my mom, sorry that I may have scared her.

I waited for her reply, but all I heard were sobs.

Finally, she managed to answer, "I love you so much; you'll never know just how much."

I woke up a couple of hours later and saw my phone on my stomach. Crap, had I hung up on my mom? I couldn't remember the rest of our conversation. I think I hung up.

Later, I called again. Dad answered the phone. "Joe, are you okay?" he said, obviously startled out of his sleep.

"When are you coming back here? Put some pep in your step!" I said.

"It's three a.m., Joe. Go back to sleep," my dad laughed. It was so good to hear him laugh.

"Dad, of all the times for you to learn to ride a unicycle, you choose now... Hurry up!" I said, hearing my dad's chuckle turn into a belly laugh. I was still confused about the time. I could have sworn the clock did not say three a.m.

I woke up. I looked at the phone in my hand. Crap! I fell asleep again!

FAMILY TIME

(ERICA)

"MOM, I'M SO worried about him. I don't know how to handle this anymore," I said. "What if he can never walk again?" My anxiety was at an all time high.

"He's going to be fine. We need to pray and ask God to look over him. We have to be strong. Don't let him see you cry!" Mom said, adamant that Joe must never see us worry. I knew she was protecting him, but this was not easy for me to do. I was so worried it was hard to contain my feelings.

It was important to keep him positive. I wanted him to feel that everything would be okay, but I just couldn't stop crying. I wanted my best friend with me. Two weeks before, we had talked about celebrating his birthday, but his birthday was nothing like we had imagined. Every morning since this had happened, I had awakened feeling like knives had pierced through my body, pinning me to my bed. To muster the strength to get up, I had to pull out the knives, one by one. I'd walk to my bathroom and stand in front of the mirror, staring at myself. I could barely recognize my brown eyes. It hurt to keep them open. They were red. I didn't understand my feelings, and I still don't understand how people process seeing the people they love hurting. I knew I should be reaching out to my friends, but I couldn't. I didn't want to talk to anyone. I appreciated their words, but nobody could take my pain away. Nobody had answers. Nobody could bring my best friend back to me. Would anything be the same again? I didn't know.

"Erica! Erica! Come on, let's go," Mom said, leading me out of the car. We were heading into the hospital, our second home.

My phone went off. "Hello?"

"Boy, do I have a surprise for you guys," my dad said. He sounded excited.

"What is it?"

"If I told you, it wouldn't be a surprise! Come on. We're waiting for you," Dad said.

"Okay. We're almost there. See you soon."

"What did he want?" asked Mom.

"He has a surprise for us. Let's see what it is," I answered, unfazed.

HOPE (JOE AND ERICA)

(JOE)

AS I WAS lying in bed half asleep, I heard my Dad next to me, shuffling in his chair. He was on his phone. I was just waking up. I hadn't noticed before, but they had taken off the cuff that had gone around my left calf and ankle for a few hours.

"Oh, my God!" I heard him shout, looking at my left foot. Dad looked away and looked again, thinking the cuff was still on my leg. He took out his phone and recorded the movement.

He was excited about something, but I didn't know what was going on because I was still wandering in and out of sleep. He said he was going to talk to the doctor, and I quickly went back to sleep.

Apparently, the doctor had told my Dad to see if I could move my leg on command. When he came back into the room, I could tell he was trying not to get me too excited. "Joe, can you move your right toe for me?" he said.

I was getting really sick of these tests, but to make him happy, I did.

He asked me to do the same with my left toe. "Oh, my God, Joe!" he yelled.

"What happened? Did it move?" I felt excited.

"Yes, Joe. You did it, buddy!"

I couldn't feel my left foot or hand, so I couldn't tell whether anything was moving. I was judging it purely on Dad's reaction.

"I can't wait to show your mom and Erica. They're going to be so happy, Joe! This is an amazing sign."

I couldn't wait to show everyone what I had done, but I was so exhausted that I fell asleep. All of that excitement and effort had taken my energy away. I went back to sleep for a couple of hours.

"Dad, where are they?" I asked when I awoke, still tired. I had a fever still, but I was so excited to see my family.

"They're almost here. They're going to be so proud," Dad said.

"Hey, Joe!" Erica and Mom said in unison.

I looked at them. Again, I could see that they were trying to be strong for me, but I knew they were upset.

"How are you feeling?" Mom asked.

"I'm okay. I still have a fever, but they're bringing me medicine for it."

Almost immediately, my mom and Erica turned and stared at my dad, worried about the fever.

"It's okay," he whispered. "They have everything under control."

If there was ever been a good time to show them what I could do, it was then. "Mom, Erica, look at my foot."

As they watched, I stared down at my foot. Come on. Work with me, I urged it. Let me make them happy. Come on…

"Oh, my God!" they yelled.

Was I doing it?

"My baby!" Mom yelled, crying at the same time.

Erica and Mom rushed around to hug me. My whole family was together, surrounding me and weeping. We must have stayed like that for at least ten minutes. I didn't realize at first how much that small movement meant to them. But after the fact, in talking with them, I understood that it mended their fear and worry more than I could ever have imagined. I wasn't going to be fully paralyzed. The movement meant that I had a bit of mobility, which in their minds meant that I would be fine.

That day, my family must have recorded the movements of my foot on their cell phones at least ten times. The excitement in the room was amazing. No childhood Christmas could ever compare to the joy in the room that day. Once my family had left, I knew I needed to keep working hard, proving to them and to me what I was capable of.

(ERICA)

"TELL ME WHAT'S going on, please!" I begged my parents. "What are the doctors saying?"

"Right now, he has something called a neuro fever. They need to focus on getting that down, and then everything will be fine. Just be positive and don't worry," Dad said.

"How can we not worry?" I cried. Everything was starting to feel overwhelming.

"We can't have him worry," Mom said. "Listen, the doctors have got him this far. Everything will be okay. We just need to focus on him and let the doctor do his job."

The next few days seemed like an eternity. Dad and I sat and stared at my brother's monitor to keep track of his temperature. We held our breath and prayed it wouldn't go up. He had a urinary tract infection. At one point, Joe told my mom he couldn't take the pain anymore. Again, Joe being in pain, the nurses and doctors coming in and out of his room, the disgusting smell of the antibacterial soap, and all the beeping from the machines made my anxiety skyrocket. I didn't know how to handle any of it. And I didn't have my best friend to discuss it with because he was in that hospital bed fighting for his life. I truly felt alone.

I felt a bit better later in the day when my parents told me Joe was requesting food. He loves bacon pancakes, and I knew that if he wanted that particular breakfast, it meant that he was one step closer to his old self. The littlest forms of normalcy served as the biggest relief for me during this horrible time.

I learned a lot about life over those few days. As we grow, parents and others try to instill in us the value of empathy for others. Hopefully, we learn what it means to put ourselves in another person's shoes and try to understand a bit more about the position they are in. I never knew what real empathy was until this experience. When my brother was in pain, it felt like someone was ripping my heart out of my chest. So many times when I feel physical pain, I realize that my brother's pain was a million times worse. In those moments, I wished I could do something to relieve his pain. I knew that I would dedicate my life to making sure he was happy, no matter what.

My parents felt the same way, I know. They did everything they could, not only to take care of Joe, but to take care of me, also. I tried to make sure they focused on him so they wouldn't have anything else to worry about.

"He's got this," Dad said to remind us that this was our only option. "Let's not show any fear. We have to pray, have faith, and stay strong for our boy."

We always heard the words, but there was really nothing any of us could do but worry.

I CAN FLY!

(JOE)

"OKAY, JOE, WE need to reposition you on this bed," the nurse said as she walked into the room.

"You're kidding me, right? I can barely move, and you think you're going to pick me up and move me?" I quipped with a smile on my face, but actually, I was curious about how she'd answer that one.

"We're going to put this sling around your body and use this device to lift you."

"Wait a second! Is that thing really going to hold me?" I said as I was being lifted in the air.

"Well, it's a little late to ask that now," I heard my dad say with a snicker.

"Dad! Dad! Quick, give me my phone," I yelled as I was dangling from the ceiling.

He hustled to get it and handed it to me.

I hurried to locate what I wanted. After about 30 seconds, the room filled with "I Believe I Can Fly," sung by R. Kelly. Laughter erupted in the room. There I was, all 6'3", 220 pounds of me suspended from the ceiling, singing and dancing (as best I could). It was quite a sight. Then again, I was just doing what I knew how to do—make people around me laugh and keep them happy and positive. Life is too short to wear a frown or be sad. And I was happy to see my dad smile and laugh. Every time he shared that story, it was great to see his smile. That was a great day. Just knowing that I was able to turn something bad into something good meant the absolute world to me.

I didn't realize how much pain the next few days would bring. Everything went smoothly until my fever started again. The doctors were trying to diminish the meds. My family was there by my side, talking to the doctors all the time. I trusted that they would always have my best interests in the forefront of their minds.

I did start to worry once I noticed that they were talking to the doctors and nurses outside of my corner room in the ICU. At the time, I didn't realize how high my fever was or even what it implied about my outcome. What was causing the fever? Couldn't they just give me meds to get rid of the fever so I could get better?

I thought things were going to get easier, but I had no idea I was about to go on an adventure that evening. The doctors kept giving me medicine. My fever would drop, and then spike again an hour later. Of course, at the time, I didn't realize this was happening. That evening, they decided that they would have to step up their efforts and do everything possible to bring my fever down and keep it down. And that's when the fun began.

I found out the hard way what the next steps were. They lifted me up again with the sling, but just a few inches off the bed. Then they placed a cooling mat under my sheets and let me back down. The cooling mat must have been 20 degrees below zero; it sure felt like that. They put the cooling mat on for what seemed to me like an eternity. It was late at night, and I was freezing. I screamed, "Nurse!" and within minutes, the nurse came into the room. It was a nurse I'd never seen before. She didn't have a common name, so it wasn't easy for me to remember.

"You need to get me off of this thing. I'm freezing!"

"Hang in there. You have twenty more minutes," she said in what sounded like a Polish accent.

It felt to me as if two hours had passed, but it was probably only two minutes before I was screaming for the nurse again.

"I told you twenty more minutes," she said, her voice forceful.

I was starting to get angry. My body felt like an ice cube and I was beyond uncomfortable. I felt trapped. I was alone in the room, didn't have any mobility on my left side, and didn't know anyone around me. I felt abandoned. What if something happened to me? Then I remembered I still had my phone with me.

"Mom, I'm freezing, and they won't get me off of this stupid cold pad!" I said when she picked up the phone. "I can't take this pain anymore!" I said in a fit of rage. "Where the hell is this nurse, because it has been way over twenty minutes by now."

"Nurse!" I screamed. I'd had enough of feeling like an ice cube.

"I told you what my name was, Joe," she said in an irritated voice.

"I really don't care what your name is, to be honest. I'm lucky I even know my own name right now." My tone was nasty. "You told me twenty minutes, and I'm freezing. Turn this stupid thing off, or at least get me some socks!" I pleaded.

The nurse assured me that she would be right back with some socks. That did not happen. Once again, I began to call for her. I didn't understand how someone could do this to another person and show no sympathy. I didn't know who this lady was; all I knew is that I didn't like her one bit.

"Where are my damn socks?" I continued to scream. "Nurse, where are my socks? Are you knitting them?"

This cycle of twenty minutes on and twenty minutes off went on throughout the night. To top it all off, I had excruciating pain in my neck and couldn't move it at all. Later, I learned that this was common after a craniotomy because the blood pools in the neck and makes it extremely stiff. Of course, my nurse right then, who was doubling as my worst nightmare, decided it was time to adjust me in the bed without giving me proper warning.

The moment she began to move me, I screamed in pain. I lost my cool a bit and yelled, "You need to let me know before you start doing things like that, because I'm in a lot of pain and you need to just get your hands off of me!" That was the last thing I remember from that night.

When I woke up in the morning, Dad was walking in the room. He said, "Joe, what's going on? The nurse said you weren't being compliant."

Only three words came to my mind in response: "*I hate her!*" I gritted out in a very angry voice. I told Dad what had happened during the night.

Finally, a nurse I recognized came in and began telling me what needed to get done that day. I completely understood and thanked her for being honest and communicating with me in a nice way, unlike the monster I'd had overnight. I was finally thawing out.

ANOTHER SURGERY?

(ERICA)

THE DAY BEFORE Joe's next surgery to fully remove the AVM, I was so nervous that it physically pained me to think about it. All I could think about was how scared my baby brother must be to have to go through the pain of it all over again. I wondered how many times they would cut his head open before this ordeal was over. I realize now how crazy my thoughts were. But at the time, I had no control over how my brain wandered. I just wanted Joe to be happy.

One of my best friends, Angelina, was there for me every step of the way. She called often and checked in on my brother. We had been friends since kindergarten. Angelina knew it was a difficult time for my family and me. She wanted to help relieve the anxiety by doing something special for Joe.

"Hey, Angelina," I said, answering my phone on the first ring.

"Hey. How's Joe doing?" she asked with genuine concern.

"He's hanging in there. His surgery is first thing tomorrow."

"Okay. He'll be fine. Please don't worry. He's really strong," she said, picking up on how petrified I was.

"I know. I just want this nightmare to be over."

"I know. Soon enough. I have a surprise for Joe," she mentioned. She sounded excited.

As I listened to the details of what she had arranged, tears streamed down my face. I wasn't surprised by her amazing generosity, and I was extremely touched by her concern and selflessness in arranging such an incredible surprise for Joe.

Going through this process with Joe was eye opening. It's easy for friends to be there for you through the good times, but this was by far the most difficult time of my life, and some friends I had thought would be by my side through it all seemed to have vanished. I chose to focus instead on the people who truly cared. Angelina was the leader of that pack, and I will forever be grateful for her.

After the call from Angelina, I called my father. "Dad, you'll never guess what Angelina has set up for Joe."

As he listened, I could hear that he was getting emotional. "Wow, I don't even have words. Angelina is a great kid! I'll have the phone next to Joe for the rest of the day," he said.

We waited....

WOW!

(JOE)

I WAS LYING in bed. Dad was sitting in the chair to my right. I looked at him. "I don't understand what this surgery is about. Why do I have to have another one?"

"Don't worry. The tough ones are over. We're almost done," he said.

"I got this. I just want to get it over with already," I said, convinced that strength was the only way to get myself through this hellish nightmare.

I tried to change the subject and talk about something fun. I looked to see what was on the television. The basketball playoffs were on, but of course that channel, the one channel I needed to watch, didn't work.

Dad was glued to his phone. Finally, he said, "I'm waiting for a phone call for you."

"For me?" I asked, extremely confused as to why someone would call for me on my dad's phone.

"Just wait and see. Be patient!" he replied.

About twenty minutes later, my dad's phone rang. He picked up right away, greeting the person on the other end. I wondered who it could be.

"Thanks for calling. He's right here. I'll give him the phone," my dad said, and held out the phone to me.

Still confused, I picked up the phone.

"Hello?" I said to whoever was on my phone.

"Hi, Joe. This is John Starks."

"John Starks, New York Knicks? You've got to be kidding me. Is this a joke?" I was stunned that I was talking to John Starks.

"It's me. I was told about what you've been going through. I know you have another surgery coming up, so I wanted to reach out and send you well wishes and some thoughts of encouragement," he said. He sounded genuine.

I was dumbfounded. A person who played in the NBA had called to check up on me. I was doing my best to choose my words carefully, because I was not only on a ton of pain medication, but I was a fan of a rival team of the New York Knicks in the '90s!

"Wow! I can't believe I'm talking to you. It's amazing. John, I have to tell you that my father, who is a huge Knicks fan, is staring at me with a smirk on his face. I respected you as a player growing up, but I have to tell you something—I'm a huge Bulls fan. Boy, did you really know how to piss me off in the '90s!" I was laughing. John Starks was known for his famous dunk over Michael Jordan, my idol and favorite basketball player of all time.

John Starks laughed. We talked about basketball for a while. We talked about '90s-style basketball and how different the league had become. Hard hits were allowed, and fouls weren't called for the "wind blowing" (as I liked to put it). I asked him who he thought would be a tougher opponent, Michael Jordan or… well, I promised him I wouldn't share, but it did make us laugh.

I was still thrilled that John Starks had called me. He didn't know me. In fact, he didn't know anything about me, yet he took time out of his busy schedule to call me. It was a wonderful conversation. After talking with John for about twenty minutes, I was overwhelmed with emotion. Not only had I gotten a chance to talk to a professional athlete, but a close family friend had cared enough to arrange this mind-blowing experience for me. I needed to thank her. I called Angelina to let her know how much I appreciated it. I was happy to know that she cared about me and that she was there for my family every step of the way.

It might sound clichéd, but after that conversation, I knew that positive thinking would get me through. I'd never thought I would get to talk to a basketball superstar in my lifetime, and look what had happened.

"I got this," I said to myself that night before falling asleep.

SURGERY DAY (JOE AND ERICA)

(JOE)

I WOKE UP feeling nervous. In a few hours, I'd be under the knife again. This surgery was a big one. They would completely remove the AVM from my brain. It would be the best thing for me in the end, and if all went well, it would drastically reduce the chances of a bleed in the future. I knew it would go well, though.

The craziest part about waiting for the surgery was that I still didn't completely understand what an AVM was, and worse yet, I couldn't comprehend what that particular surgery was for, either. All I knew was that it needed to get done, and I needed to remain positive. I was concerned because everyone around me was upset. I didn't know what was going to happen. I just knew that I was alive. My family was with me waiting for the doctors to take me into surgery, which was scheduled for a nine a.m. We made small talk while we waited. Every two minutes, someone would look at the clock.

"Joe, there's an emergency right now. Dr. C has to take care of this patient before he's able to take you in. We're going to have to delay your surgery for a bit," a nurse said.

"Oh, okay. Thanks," I said. I was anxious to get it over with, but I truly hoped that the patient with Dr. C would get out of emergency surgery as positively as I had. My family was around me. I could see that everyone was aiming to distract me to keep me from being nervous, but I knew that they were even more nervous than I was. I had to keep them from being nervous.

"So, I can't believe John Starks called me!" I said, breaking the silence. "He really stayed on the phone with me for a long time. He must be busy, too."

"Does this mean I converted you into a Knicks fan?" Dad asked.

"Not a chance!" I replied. I always have been and always will be a die-hard Chicago Bulls fan. "In fact, Dad, guess who else is a new Bulls fan?"

"Who?" he asked curiously.

"Me," Mom said, a huge smile on her face.

"Oh, no! First my son, and now my wife. Erica?"

"He got me too, Dad!" Erica said. I had converted everyone except my dad into my very own Bulls fan club. We all laughed for a bit as my mom recited the starting lineup.

It was like old times. My family could get through anything together.

"We're all set," the nurse said as she came into the room. She had a few people with her. Instantly, I felt the thumping in my chest. Well, I'd gone through the worst of them; I figured I could get through this one.

My family was visibly emotional. They weren't crying, but they would begin as soon as I left. I could tell that instantly.

"You'll be great, Joe. We love you so much," Erica said, tears pooling in her eyes. I could tell she was disappointed in herself for showing me that she was emotional.

"My Joe is my hero. You'll get through this and we will be here waiting for you!" Mom whispered as she kissed me on the forehead.

"Grandpa Joe is with you. Once you're done with this surgery, I'm going to bring you the best bacon pancakes you've ever had!" Dad was trying to joke with me, but I could see that he was very nervous.

"I love you guys. Please don't be scared. I'm strong. Just another few hours and I'll be done! Please don't worry. Dad, take care of them," I said. I was very worried about me, but even more worried about my family.

"Always," Dad said, holding my hand.

As they prepared to roll me away, I kept thinking, "Come on, Joe. You got this." I knew I could do a little better than that to make sure everyone was calm and smiling. I mean, what if something happened to me? I wanted to make this moment something they would always remember. As they rolled me out of the room, I did everything in my power to make the bed bump into things. Slowly, we went through the doors, and I made sure to make a loud noise as if we had just hit a brick wall. "Doors? No one has time for doors around here! I'm Joe Slota, and I plow through any walls and doors!" I yelled while laughing hysterically and staring at my family. They were laughing with tears in their eyes. Success! I had accomplished exactly what I wanted to do. My family was laughing. I knew for at least a few minutes, the severity of what was about to happen was on the back burner, and they could enjoy the blessings in life.

"Well, here goes nothing! I got this, guys. I'll see you in a few hours. I do expect some good food when I get out of there, you know!" I was smiling, and there were some tears in my eyes that I tried to hide from my family.

(ERICA)

"I CAN'T WAIT for this to end. I can't watch them wheel him away again. It's heart-wrenching," I cried to my parents.

I didn't want to see another person in scrubs for the rest of my life. I didn't want to smell that stupid antibacterial soap anymore. I definitely didn't want the chaplain intern to try to counsel me in the waiting room again. I wanted this to be over.

There was nothing for anyone to say. We all just sat together and said a prayer for my brother. He was in good spirits, but I knew he must be nervous. My parents were confident that he would be fine. I never knew if they were really as confident as they expressed, or if they were worried about me being scared. Regardless, my brother's fate was in God's hands.

The rest of my extended family sat with us during surgery. Zia was there every step of the way. There was nothing she wouldn't do for my family. Later on, I reflected on this period of my life, and what never made sense was why things still ran so smoothly. So many little things got done, despite the fact that my parents and I did not take care of them. Now I know that Zia took care of the things we didn't even think about. She didn't ask; she just did what needed to be done. I love her for it.

As we sat in the hospital waiting room, another family walked in. They were crying hysterically and all trying to comfort one another. I knew exactly what they were going through. Although I wanted to do something to comfort them, I knew that they needed to go through the motions of this process and they needed to be with family. As selfish as it might have seemed, I couldn't watch them. Reliving the first night in the hospital was something I couldn't handle. That's when I asked my family if we could go to the Caregivers Center. They immediately agreed, and we were on our way.

The Caregivers Center at the hospital was a calming environment. It was quiet and had a few separate rooms where families could sit. They offered free coffee and food, and they had massage chairs. My family took up one of the rooms, and we started talking about our funny memories with Joe.

I love so many things about my brother. One of his greatest qualities is that he can make anyone laugh at any time. His impersonations and jokes never end. His personality is addictive. These qualities in addition to his huge heart have always made him a wonderful person to be around.

So we told stories, and in between, a silence would come over the group. I knew that all of us were thinking about how close we had come to losing Joe. In a small family, each member has a significant trait that is an important piece of our puzzle. Not only had my brother and I always been protective of one another, but we also balanced each other out. Every time he struggled in life, I was always the one to defend him. Now, there was nothing I could do but pray while he was in the doctors' hands.

"He's all good," Dr. C said in a confident voice as he walked into the waiting room. "I'm pretty sure we got it all."

"Thank God!" we said in unison as we cried in relief. In that moment, the tension that had been building over the hours of waiting slowly dissipated. It had been a huge day that could have gone very wrong, but once again God had been on our side.

"What comes next?" my Dad asked, staying focused on getting Joe better.

"In six months, he'll have to come in for an angiogram and cranioplasty" Dr. C said. Noticing that we had no clue what that meant, he explained. "Basically, we will be able to go through your son's groin with a test that uses a special dye and camera to take pictures of the blood flow going through his brain. We will also be putting the bone flap back into his skull at that time."

"Thank you for taking care of my boy. God bless you," my mom said, and hugged Dr. C.

"It's my pleasure. He's sleeping now. They'll call you from the recovery area once he's awake," Dr. C replied.

WAKING UP AGAIN

(JOE)

WOW, I WAS in pain. Where the hell was I? Who was talking to me?

"Joe, it's Dad and me. You're okay. We're here," Erica said.

"You did a great job. They got it all," my Dad said. He sounded excited, but I could sense that they were crying.

"I'm sorry, guys. I'm sorry that I'm putting you through all this. I hate it. I know how much everyone worries," I cried. I couldn't stand the thought of my family waiting for hours to see if I would be okay. I could only imagine how worried I would be if I were in their shoes.

"Don't you dare apologize," Dad said. "We're a family, and that's what families do. We love you, and there's no place any of us would rather be than right here with you."

I could tell he was serious. Erica just looked away. She had on that face that I know so well. She was trying to gain her composure so I wouldn't notice she was crying, but I know her better than that. I couldn't help but continue to cry and apologize to them. I absolutely hated that they had to see me like I was. This thing needed to be over already. I needed to show them that I was bigger and better than my situation. I would overcome it and prove to them that anything is possible. I would never make them worry again.

After each member of my family came in to visit, I knew I needed to rest. I was in pain and wanted to sleep as much as I could. I was physically and emotionally exhausted to the maximum.

Over the next few days, I worked hard to regain my strength. I moved my left arm and leg as much as possible. Although I was in and out of pain, I wanted to get out of the ICU and into rehab as soon as possible. The only way that would ever happen, in my opinion, was to prove to them that I was physically ready.

Soon, the doctor said I could have more visitors. I was thrilled that I would see my friends. Before they arrived, I went for another ride in the sling. Once again, I sang as I was moved from the sling to the chair. It was a big event for me, because it would be the first time since the event that anyone outside my family would be able to see me sitting upright in a chair.

I visited with my friend Anthony for a while. He asked me to be the best man at his wedding. I was honored that he asked to be there for him on one of the most important days of his life. My friend Dave came by to visit also. Seeing everyone's reactions was great. I looked damn good for someone who'd had a few major brain surgeries.

I sat in the chair feeling like I was sitting on top of the world. Meanwhile, I was oblivious to what was going on outside of my room. Little did I know we were going through a heat wave and the power had gone out. Dave was telling me how hot it was, which explained why he had walked in looking all sweaty. The ICU in the hospital was functioning on generators. I felt cool enough because I had a cold washcloth on my head to relieve my headaches. My family took turns making sure the washcloth was cold.

I was in excruciating pain while they were weaning me off the medication I was on. All I wanted was to hang out with everyone without the pain. I would have given anything to feel like me again. As I engaged in conversation, I got tired, and suddenly a terrible migraine came on. I couldn't control it. I appreciated the opportunity to see my friends, but I had to be honest. I couldn't hang. I was in too much pain and just too damn tired from sitting up. My friends noticed that I was struggling and left shortly after. I had been happy to see them. It was a step in the direction of normalcy.

During the next several days, I quickly began to recover and get back to myself. I was slowly coming off the heavy medication. I was given methadone to wean me off it without suffering withdrawal.

When they first told me I was being given methadone, I said, "I'm not going to be walking around like a crackhead, right? I've never taken a drug in my life."

Everyone laughed when I said that. The nurses assured me that I would not look like or become a drug addict. I wanted to be sure of that, so I tried to limit my requests for heavy pain meds. I could deal with the pain. I had survived so far. The worst was behind me. Looking back, that probably wasn't the smartest decision I've ever made in my life.

The day before I left the hospital, I had a very important moment with my mom. Every minute of every day, I sat in my bed, practicing moving my fingers and my toes. I was eager to make my family smile instead of seeing them worry. I wanted them to know that I was ready and willing to face whatever lay ahead of me.

"Hey, Mom. Come here," I said. She walked over. "Put two of your fingers in my hand," I said, indicating my left hand. She did as I asked. I squeezed both of her fingers. My entire left side had been immobile just days before, but this was a sign that my strength and further mobility were coming back.

I waited for her reaction. She started crying and hugged me as tightly as she could. I was proud of myself, but I didn't realize the extent of the pride my mom had in me until that very moment.

DISCHARGED TO KESSLER (JOE AND ERICA)

(JOE)

DAD CAME INTO the room with my breakfast. The smells of food and hand sanitizer were overwhelming.

"I have great news," he said, sounding proud. "The doctor just told me that you've been doing very well, so today you're going to Kessler to start the next phase of your recovery."

It was the best news I had heard in a long time. I was scared at first, but I realized I had to face my journey head on. I needed to be strong. I mean, how hard could it possibly be?

As the day went on and I waited for the transport from Overlook to Kessler Institute for Rehabilitation in West Orange, New Jersey, I joked around with the nurses, who had become my friends. I asked for pictures with all of them and promised them I'd be back to visit. I had to come back and thank them for all that they had done for me. It took some time for the transport to get to the hospital. I tried to make the best of the situation. I figured if I was going to be discharged from this place, I might as well go out with a party.

After a few hours of joking around and laughing, the news came that transport was ready and I'd be leaving in twenty minutes. When they brought the stretcher up, I decided that was the best time to play my exit soundtrack. I put on Michael Jackson's "Don't Stop 'Til You Get Enough" as they wheeled me out of the hospital. All the nurses walked alongside the stretcher. They danced and smiled while the music played. I remember seeing the line of professionals in scrubs, dancing around, and just thinking to myself how amazing it was to meet such great people, even under these circumstances.

Being outside for the first time in a long time was an interesting feeling, even though it wasn't for a long time. The toughest, longest, and scariest hospital stay of my life was coming to an end. It was bittersweet. The next phase of my battle lay ahead. I was a fighter. I wouldn't give up until I knew I was successful.

"Here goes nothing," I thought as I watched the ambulance doors shut and got ready for the ride. "I hope they let me play with the sirens," I thought.

When I was brought into Kessler, I was still thinking I'd get through it and go back to living my life as I had before June 9th, 2013.

They rolled me into my room via wheelchair. I figured this was standard protocol and thought nothing of it. I would be sharing the room with a gentleman whose name I have since forgotten. We engaged in small talk for a while. At first, I was uncomfortable being out of my hospital environment without understanding the full reason I was there and wondering if I would get the same treatment I'd gotten at the hospital. If I was in pain, would I get immediate care, as I did at the hospital? How come I didn't see nurses everywhere? Why was it so quiet compared to the hospital? These were just some of the million questions running through my mind. I felt really alone and scared. I knew I wasn't allowed to get up out of bed, but I didn't know that I couldn't even if I tried. That feeling alone was really scary. If I had to use the restroom, I was stuck with an empty plastic container next to my bed. I felt as though all of my independence had been stripped from me completely.

My parents came into the room to see me shortly after I arrived. Once they were there, I felt a little more at peace. We talked and joked as if nothing had happened. Since the big event, I had felt it was my job to show the world that I could overcome what had happened and do it with a smile. I took pictures with my family, all holding hands and giving a thumbs up, which I posted on social media to inform friends that I was fine and that nothing was going to get in my way.

Once I was settled in, the doctors and nurses paid me a visit to go over the medications I would be on and then gave me a rundown on my schedule of occupational therapy, speech therapy, and physical therapy. Clearly, they would keep me busy during my weeks there. It was really overwhelming, but I knew that it had to get done.

Over the next several hours, the rest of my family came to visit. It was an emotional time.

Alone again, I was trying to get some sleep. My roommate complained of pain and kept yelling for the nurse. I have always hated hearing or seeing people in pain, so I hit my call button to get a nurse into the room. When the nurse came in, I told her that he'd been screaming in pain for the last half hour and I wanted to make sure he was okay. The nurse said that she would check on him and for me to try and get some sleep. I told her I'd try and would call if I needed anything.

The period of calm lasted about fifteen minutes before my roommate was complaining again and calling for the nurse. I felt horrible. I had no clue why he was there, and I didn't feel it was my place to get into his business and ask him. I told him that I'd called the nurse again and that things would be fine. The nurse came back, but she came to me first. I told her I was nervous being in the room with someone who was in so much pain. I explained that I'd love to help however possible, but I was not allowed to get out of my bed.

"That is very sweet of you, but we will ensure that he is in good hands."

I felt reassured that he was going to be okay when he told the nurse, "I'm cold."

All that screaming and complaining for that? Well, I was glad it was nothing serious, at least.

"You really need to get some sleep. You have a long day ahead of you."

Quietly, I mentioned to her that I would have a hard time sleeping if he kept screaming and asked if there were any private rooms available.

I've never been one to complain, but I had gotten yelled at for not getting as much sleep as I needed while I was in the ICU, and I knew a private room would be best for my recovery. Luckily, they had one available and were able to transfer me a few hours later.

(ERICA)

ONE OF THE most difficult parts of this journey was when I found out that my brother would be going to a Kessler only two weeks after his first surgery. I did not think he was ready for it. He was progressing quickly, and I had expected that he would not leave the hospital until he was 100 percent back to himself. I was nervous. I received the call that he would be leaving the hospital from my parents while I was at work. That day was horrific. My coworkers consoled me, but nothing they could say or do could make the experience any easier. I prayed that Kessler would work hard to get my brother walking again. He still had limited mobility on his left side. His vision was not back fully, either. I questioned my parents after every trip to the hospital because I refused to ask them anything in front of Joe. But I wanted to know.

Why was he talking so slowly?

Why was his voice so high-pitched?

When could they put his bone flap back in?

I had many questions beyond those, but the only answer was time; time would reveal how much he would progress. I thought I was a patient person, but I couldn't wait for the answers. I wanted to know them *now*.

On the day of Joe's transfer to Kessler, I begged my parents to ask the staff if he could stay in the ICU for a bit longer. The nurses there had become family to us, and I was more comfortable with their care for Joe than with people I had never met. My expectations were extremely high, and they had gone beyond anything I could have imagined. You meet people all the time and forget their names and faces. I will never forget any of the care team at Overlook for as long as I live. They treated my family with empathy and respect.

After work, I drove straight to Kessler. I wondered about the procedures for getting into the hospital. Would I have to get permission to see him? Would they let me right in?

I sat in my car for ten minutes, looking at old text messages between my brother and me. (I have a habit of keeping text messages for a long time.) I read the conversations from June 7th and 8th. My brother had texted me as he normally would, sending jokes. I smiled at first, and then I cried. I realized how lonely I was without Joe. He was there physically, but emotionally and mentally, I didn't know if he would ever be the same. Had I lost him forever? Tears streamed down my face. I was sad, but I was also mad at myself because the tears delayed my visit for a few minutes. I couldn't let him see me cry.

"What's taking you so long? Let's go! Put some pep in your step!" Joe texted me.

His text turned everything around. I had needed him to say something he would normally say, and he had done it at the very time I needed it. I wiped my tears and told myself that I could do it.

I stepped outside and felt the summer heat on my face. I went to the front desk, where a man in a wheelchair greeted me. At first, I wondered if he was a patient. Then he welcomed me and asked me who I was visiting as he wrote out my name badge. I was impressed with how kind and professional he was. I was happy that the first person I encountered in this new place was welcoming. It made me feel like Joe was in good hands.

Those elevator rides up to the third floor were always interesting. I would get myself into gear and prepare myself. On this first visit, Mom was waiting for me outside the elevator. I hugged her. I needed my family more than I could ever have expressed. I was being as strong as I could for them, but my strength was dwindling every day. I asked her how Joe was. She said he was absolutely fine and had been making everyone laugh all day. That was Joe. Of course he would make light of the day.

Joe's first day at Kessler gave the nurses and doctors an opportunity to evaluate him. They got a full picture of what he had gone through and were working on a good plan to help him recover as quickly and fully as was humanly possible. The nurse estimated that Joe would be at Kessler for roughly two weeks. Again, I was uneasy with this timeline. I didn't want them to skip any steps or hold him back from recovering to his full capacity. I voiced my concern to my parents, and they assured me that they were on top of it.

FIRST STEP (JOE AND ERICA)

(JOE)

IT WAS EARLY on the morning of my first day of therapy. When I opened my eyes, all I wanted to do was go back to sleep. With the medications and not having to be on a schedule for a couple of weeks, it was overwhelmingly difficult to wake up so early.

My father came into my room with breakfast. I found it difficult to eat because I didn't know what therapy had in store for me. When I was helped into my wheelchair by one of the nursing assistants at Kessler, I was a little confused. I thought I was in the wheelchair because of protocol. I thought it was odd that I couldn't just walk into therapy. I figured I would be going into the gym for strength training. After being in the hospital for so long, I thought it was just that my muscle mass had declined and all I had to do was build myself back up. I was unpleasantly surprised.

I strapped on my beautiful helmet, which was given to me at the hospital to protect my head because a piece of my skull had been removed. My father and the Kessler nursing assistant rolled me into the gym for therapy. It was a feeling I will never forget. The moment they rolled me through the doors, all I saw were many people who needed help. Some struggled to speak and some weren't moving much; others had tubes coming out of their throats. It was scary. Someone had to help those people. I used my right arm to try to stand up to see if I could help them. My father and the nursing assistants wouldn't allow me to get out of my wheelchair to help. I was confused as to why. I hadn't known what I was in for.

A few minutes later, my therapist came over to me.

"Hi, Joe. I'm Jenna. I'm going to be your physical therapist."

We sat and talked for a few minutes about my goals. I had to do some initial testing. She mentioned they would test my balance and walking ability. I was a bit nervous. I was 6'3", and balance had never been my forte.

Jenna called one of her therapy assistants over to help. The assistant, Morris, introduced himself to me. They also brought over what looked to be an extremely large walker. It had wheels at the bottom. They stood on either side of me and helped me stand up from the wheelchair. It felt great to stand.

"Joe, we're going to hold your arms and keep you up. You have to trust us. We're not going to let you fall," they said.

With my right foot, I took a small step forward. I was about to continue my forward motion with my left foot, but I started to tip forward. In my mind, I thought my left foot had moved forward and would be in place. When I looked down, though, I saw that my leg was just dragging behind me. I'd had no idea I couldn't walk. It hit me like a ton of bricks. I felt my heart in my throat and tingles throughout my body. What the hell was going on?

I didn't have full sensation, so I couldn't tell where my left side was in space. Once they realized my lack of mobility, they decided I'd have to use the walker. They told me to place my arms on top and to use the strength I had to hold myself up. I had only taken one step, and I was sweating profusely. I didn't have a clue as to what was going on. I attempted to take another step with the walker, and my leg continued to drag. I remember thinking to myself, "Come on Joe. You've done this your whole life. It's just walking, nothing new."

They continued to help me try to walk with the walker. My left arm kept falling off the walker because I couldn't feel whether it was lying on top or dangling by my side. They recognized that this was an issue, so they strapped my left arm to the top of the walker. As I took steps, they guided my left leg in the forward motion. It was a deeply frightening experience. I had been planning to play basketball in the fall.

We continued for the remainder of the hour.

I hadn't realized how much of a workout it would be to take a few steps. I was drenched, and the helmet didn't help the situation much. It took everything inside of me to take those first steps. It was at this point that it occurred to me that I was in fact one of the individuals who I was trying to help. I'm one of them. This was a very emotional and overwhelming feeling that took over me. I tried my best to hide it from everyone, but I'm sure I was anything but successful.

When I was done with physical therapy, I got a bit of a break before I moved into occupational therapy. The staff rolled me to a different part of the gym where the therapist would prepare the equipment for my OT. They did initial testing to identify the mobility of and sensation in my left arm. I hadn't thought it would be as much of a struggle as it was. One exercise was to take large pegs and fit them into large holes. When they first set that in front of me, I laughed. I remembered it from preschool. I picked up my left arm and reached for the peg. I knocked the bucket over.

What the hell was going on? I had been able to move my arm in the hospital. What about the strength training? That pegboard was difficult.

The therapist picked up the pegs and put them back on the table. She reassured me and said I could try again.

In the meantime, another patient was screaming and cursing. I struggled intensely with every exercise I had to do, including taking my sweatshirt on and off: I couldn't figure out how to do it. My mind was telling me what to do, but something filtered or blocked the logical next step to completion. It was frightening. I felt trapped in my own head.

Next, I was instructed to draw a clock with the numbers. I didn't expect it to be a problem. But I am left-handed. Just holding the pencil was a chore. I drew the circle, or so it was supposed to be. Since I couldn't get much of a circle drawn, they gave me a sheet with a circle on it and told me to write in the numbers. I couldn't get the numbers in the right locations spatially. It was like thinking through a fog. It should have been so simple. Why couldn't I do it?

My eyes filled and tears rolled down my face. I tried to hide them. Why had this happened to me? Would I ever be the same again?

"Come on, Joe, man up," I urged myself silently. "You can do this." I was not going to allow another tear to be shed. I knew nobody else could do the work for me. I couldn't give up. I was lucky I was alive. God had kept me here for a reason.

I looked over and saw my mom's face. She smiled, as if to comfort me. I never wanted to see that smile off my mother's face again. It was her smile that comforted me. If that was what she intended, she was successful. I vowed I would keep that smile on her face.

I endured through the rest of my OT therapy for the day. I asked the therapist what I could do in my room to accelerate my recovery. She mentioned that I could squeeze a stress ball or touch each finger to my thumb in order and back again. However, she would prefer it if I rested.

I'd have those hand exercises perfected by the next day, I was sure. I left that session sweating profusely, too. You would think that I wouldn't sweat performing activities that weren't intense, but my mind was working in overdrive to recover, and that is what caused me to sweat.

My last therapy session for the day was speech therapy. I seriously felt like a four-year-old when they started the initial testing.

The therapist held up flash cards and asked me to identify numbers and letters in order. Were they kidding me? I could have done that stuff in my sleep. I didn't understand why it was making me so tired. I didn't understand why it was so difficult to locate numbers and letters on a card. I was confused about what was going on. I got frustrated and overwhelmed all at once, and I couldn't control my emotions in the slightest bit. I was all over the place! I'd feel extremely happy and then extremely sad. I was exhausted. Thankfully, speech therapy ended just in time, because I didn't think I could take another minute of it.

After therapy, they took me back to my room to rest. The neuropsychologist came in and talked to me about some medications I would be on and asked if I had any questions. I asked why they had me on an antidepressant; I wasn't a sad person, and I didn't want to become dependent on a drug.

Her response was interesting. Studies had shown that the lowest dose of this particular antidepressant could help with fine motor skills. I agreed to take it. She also told me that my senses were heightened, and my emotions would be extreme, both good and bad. How right she was! My emotions were taking me on a rollercoaster ride that I didn't want to be on.

(ERICA)

AFTER LEARNING ABOUT Joe's first day of therapy, I knew he was safe. I continued moving Joe's fingers and helping him with whatever exercises they thought would be beneficial. I was optimistic about his physical recovery. I worried most about his cognition. As a trained counselor, I was aware that he would likely be given a battery of tests to measure his current cognitive level. I wanted to participate in that.

I sat in on Joe's first meeting with his speech therapist. She was intelligent, and she was very good with Joe. I listened to every word that came out of her mouth. I didn't want to miss anything. She tested him with flash cards and asked him to recite some letters and numbers. She also gave him a memory test, which he performed very well on.

After their session, I sat down with her and told her I wanted to know everything. She looked at me a bit oddly at first, but after staring into my eyes for a good five seconds, I think she understood that being able to work on the exercises with Joe meant a lot to me. She took the time to review his homework with me.

Joe had problems with his vision. It was difficult for him to decipher the first word on the left side of a sheet of paper. I could assist by practicing scanning and highlighting with him. It made me think of our college years. Joe and I had taken a few classes together. I always took a ton of notes, studied hard, and finished up my papers quickly. Joe was just the opposite. He listened in class but I never saw him take any notes. Somehow, though, he always did well on his assessments despite his lack of enthusiasm and effort in the classroom. I worried about this because I didn't know if he would continue the same bad habits during this critical time in his recovery.

After the therapist left, I sat with Joe for a bit longer. I went through some of the exercises she had given us.

As Joe practiced, he got frustrated with the work. "Erica, why is this happening?" he said, tears in his eyes.

"Joe, just take a deep breath and try your best. You just went through major brain surgery. You'll get the hang of it," I said. I hoped that my encouragement would be enough to keep his morale high.

For the next hour, we went over all the exercises we could. I was determined to do all I could to make sure that my brother's mind recovered to be just as sharp as it had been before his surgery. I couldn't let him down. I wouldn't let him down. At the end of the hour, I decided we needed to talk.

"Joe, you are smart, and I am so proud of you. There is not a thing in this world that you can't do. I love you with all of my heart, and I promise that I will give all that I can to make sure you get through this. It's always been us as a team, and that is not going to end now.

Keep your head up," I said. My tears flowed. Joe looked at me and I saw his eyes fill up.

"Please don't be upset. I'll do it, I promise," he replied, clearly trying to make me feel better. I hated getting upset in front of him. There were times I could choke back the tears, but then there were times when it was impossible.

"I'm not upset. I'm crying because I'm so proud of you. Look how far you've come in such a short time. Joe, you're going to leave here stronger than ever. I have no doubt about that. I just need you to be as positive as you can. I don't want you to worry about Mom and Dad. I'll take care of them. Just focus on your recovery."

Joe didn't have to say a word. I knew he was worried about all of us. I could feel in my bones that he was scared and frustrated. I knew he wanted to be there for us, but he had to focus on himself. I had to be strong. I had to find the strength in my mind to take care of my family and not show them how terrified I was. I had never been more scared in my life.

I had a few close friends who checked on me every day. Besides my family, those people kept me going. They seemed to know when I needed to talk and when I needed to be distracted. I will be forever grateful to the friends that stuck by my side and never let me down. And as can happen in most difficult situations, sometimes you lose close friends. Often, people don't know what to say or how to react when you are going through something difficult. Of course, at that point, I didn't hold anything against them. I was too focused on my family to care. It wasn't until further down the line that I realized how important it was to focus all my efforts and love on the people who were there rather than holding ill feelings toward those who couldn't or wouldn't find the time.

On that day in rehab, I realized that my brother had become my hero. The doctors might have saved his life, but he had saved mine. Had he lost his life, I wouldn't have been the same again. I couldn't give up on him. It wasn't an option.

Leaving Kessler that night was difficult, but I was strong. I spent my evening researching cognitive exercises and finding things that Joe could do when he was resting at Kessler. I knew he'd be busy, but I wanted him to feel as comfortable as he could. Summer had started for me, and I planned to focus all my time and energy on being with Joe.

CAR AND PEGS

(JOE)

I'VE NEVER BEEN a morning person. Every morning I woke up to the sensation of a doctor or nurse gently shaking my chest. "Good morning, Joe. Time to go to therapy." I opened my eyes to a new face every morning. For a moment, I'd be shocked and disoriented, wondering where I was. On some mornings, I got a little upset. I prayed I would wake up and be at home in my own bed, feeling relief from a horrible dream. I'd be awakened at about 8:45 a.m. and had to be ready for my therapy session at 9 a.m. It took me a while to shake my crankiness, but once I realized where I was going and what I had to do, I geared up to take on my problem headfirst and speed up my recovery.

Every morning, my dad walked through the door with a bag in his hand. Usually, it was a bagel with cream cheese and smoked salmon. As I took my first bite, I'd smile and tell Dad and the nurse, "I hope nobody has to get too close to me today. My breath is going to be kickin'!" They'd crack up laughing. Not wanting to be late for therapy, I'd say, "Let's get the show on the road!"

Dad would wheel me to the gym while I finished my breakfast. My occupational therapist usually came over, as I was texting on my phone. "How many times do I have to tell you—no texting during therapy?" Of course, every time, I'd give a smart-ass comment, something along the lines of, "Don't hate me 'cause you ain't me!"

One day, the therapist said we'd be practicing something new. I liked that. I was in favor of pushing myself to new limits. Then she mentioned we would practice getting in and out of a car.

"Really! I can't wait to drive again. Will that come soon?"

Her reply hit me hard. I saw her disappointed look. "Joe, that might not happen for a very long time."

I had been thinking that I'd be back to "normal" in a few more weeks.

"No," I said, "I'll be driving soon."

To ease the situation, she said, "Let's practice this next exercise. It's the first step to getting there."

She wheeled me to the back of the gym to where there was an imitation car. "Okay, Joe. We're going to practice getting out of the wheelchair and sitting in the car," she said. "Let's be really careful. I'll teach you the proper way to do this so that you don't hit your head. We don't need any accidents, now!" she joked.

I knew I had to be patient and careful. It was early in the morning, so I was exhausted. The movements took a toll on me physically. I kept relying on my right arm. When I first stood up, I felt as though I had been sleeping for three weeks. I held on to the side of the car while the therapist was behind me, supporting me. I stretched. Even that was a difficult task for me. If I leaned a little too far to one side, I lost balance.

"Give me a heads up before you stretch, so you won't fall."

She taught me how to sit in the car. "You're going to turn around, sit first, and then swing your legs in," she said, making sure the directions were clear.

Apparently, my days of just plopping in the car were over. Time to break that habit. We practiced for a few minutes. Then I did my typical walk around the gym with assistance. We had practiced walking like this over the previous several days, and I was getting a little better. My baby steps motivated me to work harder.

The next part of my therapy focused on my arm and hand. Tasks that used to be so simple had become challenging. My therapist brought a board and pegs; these were different from the ones I had used in the initial exercise. This board had many small pegs in it. My task was to remove the pegs and put them back in using only my left hand and keeping my right hand behind my back. While working through this activity, I got very frustrated. The amount of brainpower and energy it took to use just my left hand fatigued me. I was sweating profusely.

Remembering they had said it would take me a while to drive again, I kept telling myself, "This is part of the process. Just follow the process." I thought about my family and the support they were giving me. I needed to prove to them that I could do it.

A few more exercises, and my therapy was a wrap for the day. It was time to go and relax with my visitors. Without fail, family and/or friends visited me every day. In fact, I felt like the mayor of Kessler! I became friends with all of the caregivers and employees. The place had begun to feel like home.

But therapy had really tired me out. Soon, I asked my father to take me back to my room for a bit. I needed to take a nap. My energy had been depleted after just an hour of conversation with various people.

As I lay in my bed trying to fall asleep, I reflected on the activities of the day. It still shocked me that small tasks had become so complicated and exhausting. I could think of only one thing, and I repeated it to myself constantly: *Everything will come back. It has to. I have big plans for my life, and I won't let anything get in the way of achieving them. Anything is possible if you want it badly enough.*

I repeated those words to myself constantly. I thought of them when I woke up, while I was working hard in OT and PT, and before bed. Anything is possible if you want it badly enough.

SOCCER, FRIENDS, AND INDEPENDENCE DAY (JOE AND ERICA)

(JOE)

IT FELT LIKE old times with family around. Italy was playing a world cup qualifying game that was going to be televised. I asked Mom if the entire family would want to watch the game in the day room at Kessler. It wouldn't be a traditional game if I didn't have my Italia jersey on. I was all set up in my wheelchair with my entire family around. I was uncomfortable. It felt like my tailbone was going to cut through my skin. Since I didn't have full sensation on my left side, balancing was difficult. My mom reclined my wheelchair back a bit to make me a little more comfortable. Discomfort wasn't going to stop me from enjoying the game.

"Mom, does the screen look weird to you?" I asked as we were watching the game. I felt like I had double vision or was going cross-eyed. I hoped it was the television.

This was the first hint I got that I had lost half of my vision to the left in both eyes, and then I figured it would come back in time with some healing. I had heard of something called "left neglect," which, to me, meant that in time my vision could be restored. I kept positive. I told everyone it would come back because, in my mind, it had to.

Italian soccer was a big part of my upbringing. As far back as I can remember, Sundays were filled with Italian announcers screaming, "Goal!" When we were kids, my sister and I played soccer with my grandfather. We even got to experience the 1994 World Cup in New Jersey. As I watched the game in the day room with my grandfather and my cousin, Luke, we talked about the players and Italy's chances in the next tournament. It felt like old times. Yes, I was struggling with my vision and trying to grasp the extent of my injury, but there was nothing like being with my family and enjoying the present, especially with an Italian victory. It was a successful afternoon.

On the Fourth of July, I felt a bit odd. Typically, I had big plans with friends to celebrate Independence Day. Clearly, this year was going to be a little different. I felt bad that my family was stuck in a rehabilitation hospital with me, and that I couldn't be with my friends. The last thing I had ever wanted was to burden anyone by making them spend the holiday at Kessler.

I finished therapy that day and headed to my room to take a shower. After I had dressed for the remainder of the day, my dad told me that some people were there to see me. Because it was a holiday, I was curious. Who was around and willing to come see me? No plans had been made for anyone to visit.

I turned toward the door and saw my friends Dave, Anthony, and Jose. I was shocked that they all had decided to spend their Fourth of July at the rehab hospital with me. I had always known I had good friends, but on that day, I realized how amazing my friends were and how much they cared. It was a good feeling to know that people cared about me enough to devote some of their time to put a smile on my face, even though it wasn't in the most ideal place.

We hung around for a while. We caused a bit of a scene in the day room, transforming it into a party area for my visitors. The staff had to lug in ten or twenty extra chairs just for my friends and family alone. We sat around and joked. It felt good to laugh. Shortly after they left, my friend Eddie came by.

Feeling that people cared for me made me want to work even harder. I wanted to make them proud, to prove to them that I could do it.

(ERICA)

SEEING JOE, MY grandfather, and Luke watch the game made me very emotional. A few summers before, the three of them had watched soccer together on TV down the shore. Now, my brother was in a wheelchair. I could tell he was uncomfortable. My cousin and my grandfather were similar in that they repressed their feelings in front of the family during this horrible time in our lives. Seeing them on either side of my brother, watching the game like old times, made me realize that the game gave them a way to let their feelings out. They needed some sort of outlet, and yelling about Italian soccer was it.

I watched from afar, studying them. My grandfather and Luke stared at my brother sometimes, each having an emotional moment within his own mind. Yes, it was sad to see Joe sitting there in a wheelchair. Yet, I was happy. I was happy to see how diligently my brother worked to keep himself propped up in that chair. Despite the level of difficulty involved, he proudly spent time with Luke and my grandfather. It is a moment that I will remember for the rest of my life.

I hadn't even thought of making plans to go out somewhere on the Fourth of July. I was focused on being with my family. The thought of my brother celebrating a holiday without any of us around was unfathomable. And when I found out that Joe's friends would be coming around to visit, I was thrilled. I thought that my brother had great friends, but knowing that they wanted to be there for him on a holiday made me feel extremely proud—of them and of Joe. They were loud, laughing, and just having a grand time turning the day room into their stomping ground, and I loved it. Seeing the surprise on my brother's face when they walked into the room made me the happiest person in the world. I have had plenty of fun at Fourth of July celebrations in my life, but that one will forever be the best.

It was a symbolic day, also. Independence and celebrations held deep meaning for me. Joe was regaining more of his independence every day because he was working diligently to make progress physically, emotionally, and mentally. He impressed me more every day.

MILESTONES

(JOE)

EVERYTHING HAD BEEN going smoothly. The first time I had attempted the treadmill, it was set to move extremely slowly, and I had needed a few therapists to guide me. At first, they placed me in what seemed to be a full body sling for my safety. That thing was *not* comfortable. I must have looked like I was strapped into my chute and ready to jump out of a plane. Someone watched my left side, my weak side, to make sure I didn't get hurt. I couldn't control where my left foot was spatially, but I could hear a noise each time it hit the front of the treadmill. I was almost marching. My leg stayed straight and I kind of swung it forward. Soon, I didn't need a brace and the second therapist contributed minimally to guiding my steps.

The therapists were extremely impressed with my progress in just a week's time. My response was always the same: "I have goals to meet. Give me the work to do, and I'll get it done." They just stared at me and nodded. It seemed they weren't used to hearing such a determined and positive attitude. I stood by my words, too. They knew I was determined just by the look in my eyes.

One day, after my warmup on the treadmill, my therapist said we were going to climb steps. I was used to climbing the small set of fake steps in the gym, but she had something different in mind. I would climb the real steps in the stairwell of Kessler. As she walked me down the hallway, she said I would use the banister to help me walk up and down the stairs. She assured me that she would be there to assist, but she wanted me to work hard independently.

My father was there to watch. The look on his face after my therapist explained the activity was priceless. He looked cartoon-style terrified. My size in relation to my very small therapist was a cause for concern in my father's eyes. He thought of the danger. If I fell, would she be able to catch me?

Noticing my dad's concern, she commanded him, "Wipe that look off your face and have confidence. If you believe in him, he'll be able to do it!"

My therapist told me to hold on to the railing, take a step with my right foot, and then meet it with my left. This is what I did for each step as I clung to the railing. I was very scared. When I got to the top, I felt really proud of myself. Then, I turned back around, and I felt my heart in my throat. I hadn't realized how high up I was until then.

My therapist gave me directions. "Now that you know that you can do this, you have to come down. I want you to do the same thing: Start with your right foot and meet it with your left."

I did it! I was thrilled. We did this a few times; gradually, I could hold on with just one hand. My confidence went through the roof. I realized that it's okay to be scared, but the only way to overcome the fear is to face it head on.

That was a huge milestone, and I was hungry for more challenges. The next time a therapist gave me the pegboard, I was up for it. Until then, I had hated the pegboard with a passion. It had been my arch nemesis. That day, though, the confidence I'd gained made me excited to meet the challenge, and more, to welcome it. I placed the pegs faster than ever!

My confidence grew every time I accomplished something new. I realized that tasks became easier when I was determined, and my success rate increased. What so many people have said about positivity being half the battle is true.

That day had been filled with meeting many goals. It became even more special when the doctor approached me after my therapy sessions. "Let me take a look at your stitches. I think we might be able to remove them today." She told me to go back to my room, get changed, and she would meet me in there later to remove the stitches.

After I was all cleaned up, Luke and my mom came in. I asked Luke if it hurt to get stitches removed since he'd had that experience. He said it wasn't the most pleasant feeling, but it was a relief to feel the release of pressure.

The doctor came in and asked if I was ready.

"Let's do it!" I said, ready.

She started with the staple on the top of my head. My mom actually cringed. Luke had a different look on his face. "That's awesome!" he said.

After she had removed all of my stitches, I felt such relief. What a perfect day that was!

GOOD MORNING!
(JOE AND ERICA)

(JOE)

THROUGHOUT MY ORDEAL, I usually didn't notice I had made progress until after it had occurred.

It was the middle of the night. I was lying in my bed at Kessler, texting and talking to friends and family, as usual. I didn't believe in taking any time off during my recovery. I knew if I worked hard, I would get to where I needed to be when I wanted to be there. In my bed, I texted with my right hand and squeezed a stress ball with my left hand. After a while, I swapped hands. Every night, I kept this going until I fell asleep.

On this night in particular, I noticed something was a bit different. My left arm seemed to wake up. It felt like a switch was turned on. And as I tried to stretch my left side as I did each night, I could feel more of a pull in my muscles than I had on previous nights. I texted my family: "I feel like Frankenstein, and someone plugged me back in. Everything is going to be fine. I'm coming back! I can't wait for therapy tomorrow."

The small milestones I had achieved were adding up and giving me the motivation I needed to succeed.

The next morning, I woke up on cloud nine. The therapists were ready to push me a little harder that day. They showed me the path I would walk and assured me that they would be behind me. "Start walking. We'll let you know when it's time to stop."

I walked the entire path twice before the therapist told me to stop. She wanted to talk to me. "I want you to know that you just did that entire path on your own with no assistance," she said.

This showed me the immense power of the mind. If you *believe* that you can achieve success, you clear away the mental roadblocks. Anything really is possible.

The therapists knew how much I loved dogs. My eyes lit up whenever I saw the therapy dogs. My therapist asked me if I would like to incorporate the dogs in my routine.

"I thought you'd never ask!"

The therapist instructed the dog to come to my left side so I could pet him with my left hand. "Can you feel his fur with your left hand?"

I could feel it slightly, but not nearly as much as I could with my right hand. "You can walk with the dog, but keep him to your left and hold the leash with your left hand." She indicated the path I had walked earlier that day. I loved dogs and was so thrilled to try walking the dog.

The dog moved slightly in front of me to my left, where I couldn't see him. That made me so nervous that I lost my balance. I felt myself beginning to fall. I didn't want to fall on the dog, so I did anything I could to avoid that. I landed on my left knee and rolled to my side so I could avoid hitting my head.

I was really bummed that I had fallen, and I was embarrassed. I was doing so well in therapy. How could I fall? I felt the fall set me back and made everyone think I couldn't do it. I also felt sorry for the therapist because I knew she would have to write up a report on the fall, even though it was not her fault. I tried not to show my emotions, but I was clearly upset and she knew it. I tried to change the subject and made a joke to avoid conversation about what had just happened.

Back in the gym after the paperwork was done, she said, "I don't want you to focus on this. It happened; it's in the past, and we are not going to let it happen again. There are only positive, good things to come." I was still upset, but I knew I had to continue working hard and not let the fall get to me.

After therapy, I was eating my lunch in the day room. My parents and sister were there. I received a text message from my friend Scott: "Hey buddy, you might want to check out your Facebook page. There's something on there that I think you'll want to see."

I didn't have my laptop with me at Kessler, so I asked my dad to pull up my Facebook page on his computer. My family huddled around me in anticipation. Someone had posted a video. I recognized a familiar face—Tiki Barber, former running back for the New York Giants. Tiki Barber had recorded a video, encouraging me and wishing me well. He was sending his well wishes by sending me messages from some of my friends.

I was in awe. First John Starks had reached out to me, then my friend had given me an autographed Derrick Rose jersey, and now Tiki Barber had videoed to wish me well. I teared up. I didn't know how to express how good I felt inside and how overwhelmed I was by these wonderful gestures. When I looked back on my life, sports had always been there to help me through the difficult times.

A couple of hours later, the rest of my family showed up to celebrate my cousin Luke's birthday. I couldn't wait to show everyone the Tiki Barber video. We celebrated as we always did, with many laughs and, well, of course, food. We played a few rounds of Apples to Apples.

That night, I felt it was important to have a conversation with Luke. I felt horrible that he'd had to spend his birthday at Kessler with me. He was a teenager, and that was probably the last place he wanted to be. "I'll be getting out of this place," I told him. "I'm going to drive again, and I owe you a birthday celebration. I'll make up for this birthday."

"I know you will, Joe. I had a great birthday. I got to spend my birthday with everyone that I love and care about. That's all that matters to me," he said.

My words weren't only for Luke. They were motivation for me, too. I was happy that at Luke's age, he was not only mature but had a great heart.

(ERICA)

THE DAY OF Luke's birthday celebration at Kessler made me extremely emotional. I had so many feelings. I cried because I was proud of my brother's accomplishments. I cried tears of sadness when I learned of his fall. I was excited that we could celebrate Luke's birthday together. I was proud that Joe had wonderful friends who kept pulling through and surprising him with priceless gifts that meant so much to him. Seeing Joe's face when Tiki Barber appeared on his Facebook was a joy.

I did my best to distract myself with my personal life when I was not at Kessler. I suspected that this would be a huge mistake in the end, but at that time, I didn't want to process any of my feelings. Every morning as I woke up, I could feel the yawning pit in my stomach when I remembered what Joe was going through. I hung out with people who were not particularly close. I didn't want to discuss what I was feeling, and they were not likely to ask. I couldn't be around people who had hung out with my brother and me throughout the years. It brought back too many memories, and Joe's absence was too much to handle. I just wanted to feel *nothing*. I prayed for Joe's recovery, for my family to feel no more pain, and for me to be numb to all that was churning within me.

I was a counselor, so I knew that repressing my feelings was a big mistake. Eventually, holding everything in would cause me more pain.

Even so, it was easy to be distracted, to have superficial conversations, and to talk about new episodes of television shows. These meaningless discussions helped me to forget my pain for a few minutes. I didn't want to process any of the hard things because processing would make them real. I wasn't ready for real, not by any means.

Luke's birthday party helped to create a sense of normalcy, because a family celebration without Joe was not an option. Yes, it took him a bit longer to play Apples to Apples. And yes, he didn't always notice if someone came up on his left side. But he was alive. He was laughing. And most of all, I could tell that his heart was filled with love. I couldn't ask for more.

CAT SCAN

(JOE)

ONE DAY, AN ambulance took me back to Overlook for a follow-up CAT Scan. The paramedics helped me get onto a stretcher. It was a new and different feeling to be rolled around while I was aware of my surroundings. The other times, I had been so out of it that I was not very aware of my surroundings. In the ambulance, I went to old reliable and started a discussion about boxing and sports with the guys in the back of the ambulance. We discussed some upcoming fights and cracked jokes to pass the time as we rode to Overlook. I see now that I looked to sports to deal with my emotional rollercoaster. When we arrived, I saw that my father had been following the ambulance so he could help me fill out paperwork.

At Overlook, I felt like a local celebrity. I waved and made small talk as they rolled me through the halls. Most people I saw remembered me from my time in the ICU. I got my CAT scan. It was all too familiar. Soon, it was time to head back to Kessler. It had been a nice little field trip. It was great to get away from my hospital bed and to feel the summer weather outside.

Back at Kessler, I got in my wheelchair and went straight into a celebration for the July birthdays. My whole family was there to join in for cake and coffee. We had a great time. It never felt like I was in a rehab hospital when my family was around. We could have been hanging out at someone's house or at a restaurant. We made the best of this situation, and we did a great job at that!

The following day, I received the results of my CAT scan. All was good! I had been a little worried, so it was a huge relief. I really didn't know what to expect anymore. I was mentally drained, and so I just put all of my trust and faith in the doctors. My job was to roll with the punches.

I was invited to participate in a patient focus group luncheon, where we would have the opportunity to provide the hospital's chief officer with feedback about the care and treatment, the staff, and our overall experience at Kessler. My mother went with me. We sat at a U-shaped table with some staff and other patients and their families. We were asked a series of questions. I sat back for the first few minutes. I couldn't believe some of the negative comments I was hearing, and watched how contagious it was. One person would give negative feedback, and others would pile on. This was not okay with me. I made it a point then to follow-up every negative with something positive.

At one point, I said, "It really does feel like a family here. Everyone has always been on my side, rooting for me and encouraging me to keep following the process. They push me to set small, attainable goals in order to reach my bigger goals."

As I processed what some of the other patients were saying, I noticed that the staff took in all of the feedback with open arms. I realized I had an opportunity to influence and to provide as much information and encouragement as possible. I wanted to make a difference. Well-rounded feedback is pivotal for positive growth. It was interesting to hear that everyone's experiences were different. I could clearly see the connection between a negative mindset and negative experiences. It was an eye-opener. No one can help you if you don't want to help yourself. Just being able to see this made the lunch worthwhile. It also helped that the food was pretty darn good.

Later, I continued to talk with some of the staff and other patients. We exchanged parts of our personal stories and experiences. We thanked each other for the support they had provided during the difficult times.

Positivity, friends, and support are all key motivators in getting through tough times.

BOWLING (JOE AND ERICA)

(JOE)

MY PHYSICAL THERAPIST, Jenna, ran a program at Kessler for patients who were progressing well. We could participate in outside activities to assist our integration back into society. Jenna told me about it and asked, "How do you feel about going bowling tomorrow?"

I was ready to go and eager.

The following day, we all met downstairs and a bus came to pick us up. My therapist asked me to climb onto the bus. Most of the others had to be lifted up in their wheelchairs. I met a sixteen-year-old boy who had a brain injury from a snowboarding incident. I saw that he was having a hard time introducing himself. As he struggled to get his name out, I vowed to help motivate him and inspire him to do better. The boy's father had come along, and I saw a look of both pain and admiration in his eyes. I knew then what my next goal would be. Not only would I recover, but I would also help this boy so that his father could smile again.

It had started to rain, but I didn't realize how hard it was raining until I climbed down from the bus. I got nervous. I was used to walking on the gym's flat, dry surface. This was a completely new experience for me. What if I didn't feel the moisture under my shoe and slipped? Well, I thought, here goes nothing.

"Not yet, Joe!" Jenna said. Handing me an umbrella, she challenged me to hold it with my left hand as I walked towards the door. The door was only twenty steps or so away, and I knew she had something up her sleeve. I welcomed it with open arms. She had my best interests in mind, and I would welcome all challenges she threw my way. And I did it!

We went in and got our bowling balls. My lane was next to the boy and his father. I was a little embarrassed—a twenty-seven-year-old man in a helmet bowling "granny" style. I knew it could get way worse.

Jenna told me to do different things that didn't make sense to me at the time. "Walk diagonally backwards towards the ball carrier and grab the ball as it is returned to you."

"Sure thing, boss!"

I looked over at the boy, who was wearing a huge grin. He had an assistive rail to help him. Seeing his smile made me feel emotional; I could tell that he was having a difficult time, but he was excited to be there, and his father looked happy to see him in a normal setting.

I bowled, and then I turned around and watched the boy. He got a strike! He actually laughed out loud. I joked around with him. "You're beating me so badly that you're embarrassing me!" He liked that. We talked the whole time. That day, we built a solid bond, and from then on, we joked around during all of our therapy sessions.

It had felt good to be out in society again and to have a somewhat "normal" day. Back at Kessler, we walked around the gym. I started to lose my balance but quickly braced myself by stepping diagonally backwards with my right foot. I had stopped myself from falling. I was surprised, and so was my therapist.

"Remember how I asked you to step diagonally backwards to the ball carrier when we bowled?" Jenna said.

"I see your tricks—and I love them!" Many little things that annoyed me at first proved to be critical to my recovery.

(ERICA)

I DIDN'T GO bowling with Joe that day, but I can tell you that I was really nervous. When my parents told me the plans for the day, I got really quiet. I worried that he would hurt himself, and also that other people at the bowling alley would make fun of him. I remembered seeing a special-needs event at the bowling alley when I was a kid. I had been mature enough to appreciate that such events existed, but I saw other people snickering. My mind flew right to that memory; I was petrified that it would happen to Joe.

All day, I waited at Kessler for Joe to come back. How was he doing? Was he enjoying himself? Would he feel defeated by the experience? I worried that being out in public would make him realize just how far away his recovery was. I wanted to hide. I wanted to just close my eyes, and once I opened them again, I wanted this nightmare to be over.

A few hours later, I heard voices coming from the elevator. Joe was back, and he was thrilled. He wasn't defeated or upset. He was motivated, excited, and seemed like he was on top of the world. My brother had changed. He was no longer a macho guy who worried about how he looked. He was a man who was going through a difficult time, and not only was he building himself back up, but he was working hard to motivate the people around him. I was very proud of him. My baby brother had gone through hell, but he was more resilient than any other human being I had ever encountered.

TURNING IT UP A NOTCH (JOE AND ERICA)

(JOE)

THE DAY AFTER our bowling trip was awesome. Jenna and a couple of other therapists could see how competitive I was and how motivated I was to come out of the ordeal in even better shape than when I went in.

"What would you like to do to feel some sort of normalcy in your life?"

I couldn't wait to get back to the regular gym, I told her, and of course, I wanted to play basketball again. The therapists saw that I was on a high after my bowling experience and had seen me speed walking in the hallways.

"Do you think you can do a push-up?" one asked.

"Well, there's only one way to find out, isn't there?"

I went to the exercise mat and got into the modified push-up position.

"Okay, Joe, take your time and slowly try and do a push-up."

I'm sure the last thing they needed or wanted was to see me fall flat on my face. Down I went into the push-up. It was a lot easier than

I had thought. I wanted to do more, and I did. With each push-up, I felt more energy and enthusiasm.

"Okay, Joe. You just did forty push-ups!" They were happy.

"We're not stopping with that, are we?" I said, grinning. I was happy. I was pumped. I was being challenged and beating every one of my milestones.

Next, I was given light weights to hold as I walked around the gym four times. That may seem like a small exercise, but it was a huge achievement for me, considering the condition I'd been in just a few weeks prior.

Next up was the bench press. I'd been impatient to lift weights again. This was not the typical bench press, though. They gave me a light, plastic, PVC-like pole with ankle weights strapped to both sides. I went through the benching motions with this bar. It was a lot more difficult than I had anticipated. When I lowered the bar, I noticed that my left arm fell a lot faster than my right. But I would not let this bring me down. As with everything else that confronted me, I vowed to keep working at it. With time, I knew I'd be back at the gym, working out. I felt wonderful! It was an amazing workout, and I was doing everything I was asked to do, and then some.

Before I was given my next exercise, an elderly lady asked the therapist to get my attention. She wanted to speak with me. I introduced myself and we talked for a bit while I took a break. The woman explained what had happened to her and asked if I wanted to share what had happened to me. And so I did.

She told me that she had been watching me for the past several weeks. "Is that your father?" she asked, pointing out into the hallway. I nodded. What she said next changed my life. Instantly, I understood my passion in life.

"I see how hard you've been working, and the progress you're making. I see the look in your father's eyes when you succeed. I can see that he feels what you feel. I want you to know that you have motivated me to work harder. I'm going to give it my all because of you. Thank you."

I didn't know what to say or do. No monetary reward could ever have given me the feeling I had. I felt a sense of purpose in life. I felt needed and valued. It was hard to believe what I had done for another person. This was why the AVM had happened to me. I was thoroughly convinced of it.

It was time for the last exercise of the day. I was pumped and ready for whatever would be thrown my way, especially after realizing that I had been given the opportunity to motivate and inspire with every action that I took.

Squats! Anyone who knows about lifting weights knows how much energy it takes to squat. Now, imagine doing squats after brain surgery.

"Let's get started!" I said aloud, but I was thinking that I'd better not fall over. I was ready to impress everyone around me. I'd gotten to know many of the therapists and patients around me. They had seen me at my absolute worst, and now they would see how hard I had been working to get to this point.

Okay, that was one squat...now two...and three...and twenty!

I couldn't wait to tell my family and friends what I had just accomplished. I had taken a huge step in the right direction for me. I would be back at it, and be back to doing what I loved in no time. I was drenched, but I joined them in the day room before my shower.

"Hey guys, guess what I just did!" I shouted.

They were dumbfounded. We smiled and smiled.

"I told you guys I got this," I said. A nursing assistant walked me to my room and I took a shower. It had been an extremely tiring day. The energy I typically had for a whole day was depleted in an hour or so for me. It was naptime, and I slept for several hours.

(ERICA)

IF WE HAD seen Joe monthly, it would have been easier to see his progress and be hopeful. But we were family and saw him every day, which made it difficult to recognize all of the little advances. I wanted my brother to be 100% again, and it wasn't happening fast enough for me. When he took three steps, I wished it were twenty. If he walked around the gym twice, I wished he could sprint around it 30 times. Seeing deficits in someone I loved so much was killing me inside. I wanted Joe to be happy and healthy.

Waking up every morning was horrible. I'd open my eyes and think I'd had the worst nightmare ever, and then it would hit me—the realization that the nightmare was real. My brother was not at work. He wasn't home relaxing. He wasn't with his friends, driving his car around, at the movies, or anyplace like that. He was stuck in a rehab hospital learning to walk again, missing part of his skull, and getting shots every single day. It made me sick. My eyelids were raw. I'd stare at my ceiling and wonder if I'd be able to stop crying.

The drives to Kessler were difficult. I'd blast music so maybe I wouldn't be able to think about what was going on. Then, I'd get overwhelmed and have to shut it off. I'd mentally prepare myself for the day. It was important to be positive. I had to smile even when I felt like I was dying inside. My brother looked up to me, and he needed me more than ever. I had to believe that he would make it through, or I would be letting him down.

Some days were better than others. It didn't surprise me to hear that my brother was doing push-ups with the therapists. Joe wasn't the same guy that he had been on the day before his emergency surgery. That guy had been negative at times and didn't like to take chances. His body was recovering slowly, but his attitude had already more than recovered. Now, Joe was outgoing and determined. And this is the reason he survived and is a better man than he was before.

SO...I'M STILL A GENIUS?
(JOE AND ERICA)

(JOE)

WHEN THE TIME came for cognitive testing, I was nervous. I had no clue what to expect. I worried. What if I didn't do well? Would they let me go back to work? If they didn't, how was I going to pay for my house and bills? I couldn't put that burden on my family. I was psyching myself out.

The doctors came and explained the different areas the test would cover over the next several hours. That helped, but I knew some sections of it might be difficult.

Some sections required me to write or identify objects on a page. They were difficult given that I was left-handed and had a some vision issues. The memory portion of the exam was extremely important to me because my excellent memory had been an ongoing joke with friends and family. From the time I was little, I could watch a movie once and memorize every line.

A series of words was read aloud to me once, and I was told to repeat as many as possible. The series was read again, and I repeated nearly all of them. We moved on to another portion of the test to take my mind off those words before repeating them again; this tested how long I could retain a memory. Following that, I was given a new set of words to remember. I wondered how many words they were going to give me. It was making me crazy, and I was exhausted. I thought I did a great job, but it was not over.

As the words were read aloud again, I had to indicate whether the word was from the first list or the second list.

Finally, the test was over. I was so exhausted. I felt like I hadn't slept in days.

My parents and sister were in the room with the doctors when I got my results. I had done extremely well, especially given what I had gone through only a few weeks prior.

I was lying in bed, completely fried. Only one thing was on my mind as they went through the results, section by section. I spoke up, my tone serious. "Can I just clarify that I understand everything you're saying? To sum it up, you're saying that I'm still a genius, right? I want to make sure I have witnesses for this."

Everyone laughed. I smiled and looked around. "No, but really, that's what you're saying—right?"

One doctor smiled and said, "Yes, Joe, you're a genius," with some sarcasm in her voice. I knew she was serious, and that's all that mattered.

The truth was that my processing speed had slowed down a bit, and that was to be expected given the swelling of the brain and the touching it had been exposed to for several weeks. Just like everything else, my brain would be fine if I continued to exercise it like every other muscle in my body.

That day, I extended my goals to a whole new level. I knew that I could accomplish anything physical if I worked hard at it, but I'd never had to work through a mental challenge like recovering from a concussion or stroke. I'll be honest: It was a scary feeling. Sometimes, during the day, I felt confused and in a fog. I was tired all the time. I couldn't keep up with long conversations involving many people.

It took me a little time to see who was talking. It was extremely frustrating.

At times, I lay in my hospital bed at night, looking things up on my phone to learn more about why the AVM had happened, what I could do about it, and, better yet, what my options would be after this crisis had passed. Some nights, I worried about being a big burden on friends and family. How could I ever rely on them to always be there and guide me through life? Would my friends give up on me because I wasn't the person I used to be? Wow, this was going to be bad!

Somehow, I would stop myself. These things were not going to happen. I wouldn't let them happen. "Come on, Joe," I'd prod myself. "What are you doing? You've come so far! Look at what you've accomplished with positivity and determination. Stick to your motto: Anything is possible if you want it badly enough."

If I let it, my mind would spin every night, as I lay in bed alone. I knew that. However, I also had vowed to spread positivity and hope to everyone who was struggling. I chose my own milestones as I worked towards my ultimate goals, and no one but me could do the work to reach those goals. I had an extremely supportive family and my friends who visited without being asked. I couldn't complain about a thing.

This got me thinking: What about people who are not as fortunate as I was, people who don't have close family and friends to get them out of a slump or help them when they are down? The thought upset me, and I swore I'd make a difference one day. I would let everyone know that it is okay to have ups and downs in recovery. Everyone is entitled to a bad day or night, but what matters is getting yourself up the next day and pushing yourself harder. Anything is possible, whether you think of the possibilities as miracles, religious experiences, scientific advances, technological advances, or something else. You never know what might happen to get you to where you want and need to be. I do know one thing, though: You can never expect the answers to fall into your lap. You need to be proactive; you have to work to get to where you *want* to be.

(ERICA)

I KNEW THAT Joe would need to meet and exceed specific milestones during his recovery. Sometimes I worried that if he didn't meet a particular milestone, not only would he be sad, but he would regress. Physically, he had made great strides, and his condition had improved enormously. His cognitive deficits scared me the most. I didn't know what to expect. He was able to participate in conversations smoothly. His vocabulary was up to par. He sounded wonderful. But I was anxious about what the testing would reveal.

What could have been horrible news was not horrible, at all. Joe even joked about still being a genius. Even when the circumstances were not the most wonderful, he found a way to make everyone smile. But I could read my brother very well, and I could tell that he was scared. He didn't know what to expect.

Sometimes, I'd see him scan the room, looking for me. He wanted to read my thoughts. I never let him guess. When we made eye contact, I'd tell him I wasn't scared and we would get through this together. I didn't want him to worry about anything, and I made sure that I did everything I could to make him feel comfortable and happy.

I've always been a go-to person for many people in my life, especially my brother. I helped to fix things when it seemed like nothing could be done. Yet my hands were tied. All I could do was show my support and be the best cheerleader I could be. I focused my attention on every word that came out of every medical professional's mouth. I asked a ton of questions without caring how stupid I might sound, because the more information I received, the better I'd be able to assist my brother throughout his ordeal.

THEY'RE NOT CALLED *CORE* MUSCLES FOR NO REASON (JOE AND ERICA)

.

(JOE)

EVERY DAY OF therapy was another tough workout. One day, I worked with a therapist named Kristy on exercising my core muscle groups. My mother came into therapy with me that day. Having a family member in the gym pushed me mentally to work harder. I loved to see them smile after I accomplished something. It was one thing to tell them that everything would be fine, but it was a completely different thing to show them: I actually *got* this!

My mom was not happy when I said, "Mom, they have me doing some core exercises, and they said it's okay if you want to join me and do them." She gave in. I may have begged a little bit and said please, but whatever it took. We started with some ab work and some work on the hip flexors. I could tell she wanted to kill me for pushing her to do them, but as usual, she did it with a smile.

As I looked towards the other side of the gym, I couldn't believe my eyes. The elderly lady I had spoken to the day prior was out of her wheelchair and walking with the therapists. She had said she was going to try harder, and she had kept her word. I was very happy.

"Do you want to go outside to try walking on the different types of pavements?" Kristy asked.

I was excited to go back outside to enjoy even a few minutes of the nice summer weather. We headed towards the stairs. I could tell Mom was nervous when I was about to walk down the stairs, but I told her it would be fine, that I had done this multiple times.

"I have total confidence in you. I know that you can accomplish anything you put your mind to."

"I am your son, and we both have the same stubborn mentality."

We laughed because we knew how true that was. Out in the courtyard were grassy slopes and different types of paving. I worried about getting thrown off balance, because I was still not 100% in that department. Walking on the grassy surface almost did throw me off balance, but as I continued to walk, it got easier.

We sat down to rest. I knew the road ahead of me was not going to be easy, but I was up for the challenge. I could have sat out there forever, but too soon, it was time for us to go back in. I must say, though, that although the weather was beautiful, it felt extremely hot in my big padded helmet. I was soaked!

After a shower and a short nap, I joined my family in the day room.

"You have some visitors," my dad said.

I looked up, and there were Alyssa and Kim from Overlook Medical Center, two nurses from the Neuro ICU.

I'd had some time to process everything that happened there and was eager to show them how hard I had been working to walk again. First, though, I needed to tell them one thing

"I'll never forget what you both have done to help save my life and make me feel comfortable in the process," I said, not with my usual bantering tone, but very seriously. I had seen with my own eyes how much running back and forth they did every day. The amount and quality of attention they gave me is something I will never forget.

We sat around the table and laughed about the tough times I gave them and the jokes we shared while I was there. I had a great time. It was a perfect end to the day. I felt very loved, and I was grateful to have such nice people in my life, cheering me on.

(ERICA)

AS JOE GREW stronger and his attitude remained so strong and positive, I felt more confident that this time in our lives would be temporary. He would have his life back. He wouldn't be in his current state forever. When I went with Joe to therapy, at first my focus was only on him. As time went on, though, I noticed that he was progressing much more quickly than others in that room. I felt sad for those people, but, at the same time, the fact that he was recovering quickly increased my hope that Joe would make a full recovery.

I was impressed with my parents, as well. Who would've thought that my mom would go to therapy sessions with Joe and actually work out? We all worked closely together to provide Joe with the support system he needed. I grew up emotionally through the ordeal. I saw how my family pushed every other responsibility aside to dedicate their time, energy, and attention to my brother. It was something that needed to be done. We never excused ourselves because we needed to be somewhere else. We wanted to be with Joe.

When Joe napped, my parents and I talked. We'd go over Joe's progress and discuss ideas for the next day. We noticed that Joe worked harder when we were there with him. He wanted to make us proud. So we took turns going to the sessions with him. We had learned that it was also important to take a step back and let them do their thing. We all wanted to help him as much as possible, so of course, our first instinct was protective, like grabbing his arm so he wouldn't fall. We learned to trust in the therapists, and also in Joe. He was going to get this done because he had proved to be the most resilient person I've ever met.

I worried about the effects of what we were going through as a family. I was a counselor, so I knew that repressing our feelings was the worst thing to do in a traumatic situation. We should be working together to let out our feelings. We had been so busy running around, talking to medical professionals, and spending time with Joe that we never had any downtime. Talking to each other about how well Joe was doing was helpful, but I was afraid it wouldn't be enough. The problem was, none of us wanted to reflect on the sadness we felt. I hoped and prayed that this would not be a problem for us in the future.

COMPETITION
(JOE AND ERICA)

(JOE)

SINCE I WAS a little boy, I've always been very competitive. I always—and I mean always—wanted to win. If there was a little friendly competition involved, it made me work even harder to win. Shannon, another therapist (who also knew Erica's friend Angelina) was working with me one day. Knowing how competitive I was, she asked if I wanted to do a push-up competition. I'm sure you can guess how excited I was to hear that.

Shannon got on one side of the mat, and I was set up on the other side. I didn't realize at the time, but some of the other therapists and patients had gathered around to watch the competition. The goal was to do as many push-ups as possible, and the first one to tap out would be the loser.

"Ready... Set... Go!"

I started doing push-ups, not paying attention to anyone around me. I hoped someone was counting, because I just kept going. I got to about around 15 push-ups and heard some laughing. I kept going. At 21 push-ups, I looked up. Shannon said she had tapped out over a minute before.

Morris, one of the therapy assistants, laughed. "Oh, you sure wanted to make sure you won, bro!"

I was ready for the next competition! I felt like I was on top of the world! I'd always thought that friendly competition brings out the best in you. Yes, I could challenge myself and reach my goals, but not nearly as intensely as when I made it into a game with a friend.

A few of my friends stopped by to visit that night. I was excited to brag about how hard I was working to get back to my old self. I couldn't wait to have a night out with my friends, like old times.

(ERICA)

TO UNDERSTAND JOE'S competitive side, let me rewind back to our childhood. Our video game selection was limited growing up, since the technology was not as advanced as it is now, but he mastered every game we played. If we played a game 30 times, he beat me 30 times. If we played football out front with the neighbors, Joe made sure his team won—and not by one touchdown, but by at least 21 points.

Angelina had been a friend of ours since childhood. Her kindness was something no one in her life could overlook, so it wasn't surprising to find out that Shannon, one of Joe's therapists, was friendly with her. But hearing that Joe had won a push-up contest against Shannon was confusing. At first, I was incredulous that a therapist would put him in a position like that. Then I remembered that they were dealing with my brother, who was the life of the party and the star of the show, always. If he wanted to swing from the ceiling, he would find a way to convince them to let him do it! In addition, they were in a position in which they had to empower their patients. But when I talked to Angelina and found out that Shannon had really pushed herself to win, I felt very happy. Joe was socializing with more people, and he was getting super-strong. He was going to pull this off. He would make it through that hell of a summer better than anyone could imagine.

My worry would always be there, though. Would he react negatively if a challenge proved to be too much? Would he cry? Would he yell? Would he give up? I always sat on the edge of my seat on therapy days, because I wasn't sure what to expect.

I could sense that my anxiety was getting increasingly worse. The events that my brother had gone through made me feel that I was not only out of control, but lost. I had no idea what the future would hold. I didn't know if I would have to take care of Joe for the rest of my life. I wasn't sure if he would be able to live a "normal" life once he was home. I had no answers, and as a person with anxiety, this was very difficult for me to accept and work through. I had no choice in the matter, so I had to learn how to go with the flow quickly.

THE END IS NEAR
(JOE AND ERICA)

(JOE)

WHEN I HEARD I was going to be discharged and sent home on July 23, 2013, I was very happy, and yet I was worried. Was I ready to go home? I had hoped to reach all of my goals before I left rehab, so why were they sending me home so soon? On the other hand, maybe I was doing better than I thought. I wouldn't let anything get in the way of going home to my friends and family and being on my own schedule.

I was scared inside, but I didn't let anyone see that. I could not and did not show my fear to anyone. They had been terrified about potentially losing me and about my reaction when I fully realized how bad my condition was. I vowed not to be selfish; I had to be tough and take things in stride and worry only when there was something specific to worry about. Instead, I focused on working harder than ever during the rest of my time at Kessler. I looked at my goals and raised them a couple of notches.

"Joe, you have someone here to see you," my dad said. My buddy Eddie was in the day room. I joined him and my dad there, and it was cool to see the look on Eddie's face when I walked in instead of being wheeled. He was surprised that I was walking so well since the last time he'd come by.

Times like those helped me get through some difficult thoughts. I would lie in bed and worry, despite my vow not to. Would my friends give up on me if I wasn't the same? As my dad, Eddie, and I sat in the day room and talked about cars and the usual nonsense, deep down it was killing me that I didn't know when I was going to be able to drive again.

I'd realize I was worrying and telling myself I couldn't let it bother me. All I needed to do was to follow the process and continue my recovery. I needed patience. That was funny to me, because I actually don't have any. That had been one of my strengths and weaknesses so far in life. It helped me to be aggressive when I needed to get something done, but it also caused unnecessary stress. I was learning, though. Tomorrow is never guaranteed. I knew that, now. Since June 9, 2013, I have promised myself to never take anything for granted again. I know I must live every day as if it's my last. There was nothing to be scared of anymore, ever. This was my second chance at life.

(ERICA)

I WAS NOT okay with it when I got the news that July 23rd was going to be Joe's release date from Kessler. He had just gotten there! This was all still so new. How could they just send him on his way? I was angry and frustrated. I was sitting at the front desk at school when I received this news. A cold chill went down my body. If they let him go so soon, that would be the end of his progress. He wouldn't have the same routine or round-the-clock therapy schedule anymore. I couldn't believe that they would just give up on him.

I went back into my office and got on the phone with my parents. I yelled. I told them they had to fight for him to stay longer. They had to push like hell to make sure the doctors understood that we weren't just going to let them give up on Joe like this. They were with Joe and couldn't say much in front of him, so I knew we'd have to have the conversation in person.

When I hung up, I put my head in my hands. How was I supposed to help my students when I couldn't even think for myself? My coworkers Tori and Kathy came in and shut my door. They stayed with me as I cried, and then they helped me talk through my emotions.

I just wanted him to be okay. What they said made sense. Joe would still be able to go to outpatient therapy. I could learn which exercises he needed to do, both cognitive and physical. That might make him feel more comfortable. It could also push him to be more independent, which, in turn, could make him work more diligently to achieve personal goals.

I felt much better after talking with my coworkers. I kept shaking my head and saying, "I can't believe I'm even talking about this. I can't believe this is happening."

Everything about the accident still felt unreal. I tried to distract myself as much as possible. But in the end, distracting myself made it more difficult for me to process. Now, weeks later, I couldn't believe that I was still sitting there in disbelief that we were going through this as a family.

Of course, I can't go back and change how I processed and dealt with my feelings, but I can say to anyone going through such an event that I strongly suggest never repressing or avoiding your feelings and emotions. They'll only bite you in the ass later. I had usually been careful not to express my worries to my parents, but every now and then, I'd reach my limit and push. It wasn't because I felt they were doing anything wrong, but I wanted to make sure that Joe's recovery was on point. None of us was at our best, so it was important to work together to ensure that Joe's care was both efficient and successful.

FOLLOW-UP APPOINTMENT (JOE AND ERICA)

(JOE)

THE DAY I went back to Dr. C's office for a follow-up, my parents took me. I no longer needed to get into an ambulance to be taken back and forth. I was excited, but also keyed up about what I might find out. I feared being told anything bad at my appointments. I feared the worst.

Dad pulled his car around to the front of Kessler. Mom helped me to the car. It felt odd to be back in a car. We headed to the doctor's office, which was down the road from my house. It was weird to be heading back towards the place where I nearly lost my life.

We pulled up to the office. My heart was racing, but I was ready to walk in there and show people what I was capable of. My parents helped me fill out the paperwork, and soon it was time to go in.

"Here goes nothing," I thought.

I walked into the exam room and was told to sit on the table so the doctor could examine my head. My parents were sitting to my right when Dr. C came in. As I usually do, I thanked him for saving my life. Then I started asking a bunch of questions. I was nervous about the answers I might receive.

Could brain neurons grow back? Was there anything I could do to help my recovery? Were there any supplements I should be taking? Would the scar look bad?

I rattled off question after question, and I stayed so nervous that I couldn't even focus on the doctor's responses as he took the time to answer all of my questions patiently. He then looked at my head and saw that one stitch was still there. As he pulled the stitch, he told me everything looked excellent. That was a relief. We talked for a bit. My parents asked questions, too.

One thing stood out to me during the appointment. When Dr. C asked how rehab was going, I was proud to tell him that I'd be getting released on July 23rd. I did not at all expect the words he said in reply, but it spoke volumes: "No crap?" It was a gift. I took it to mean that I was ahead of schedule and having an excellent recovery. In fact, I was on top of the world.

"Go to the front desk on your way out and schedule your next surgery to put the bone back into your head."

"Believe me, it will be my pleasure. I can't wait to get out of this helmet. Do you know how hot this thing is in the summer?" I laughed.

We set the date of my surgery for December 2, 2013.

I couldn't wait to give the great news to Erica and everyone else. On December 2, 2013, my awful journey would come to an end.

I'd be lying if I said I wasn't nervous. It was still another surgery. I'd get my head cut open and have a bone screwed back into my head. At that time, my bone was somewhere in the Midwest at a storage facility. That was difficult to come to terms with. My skull, half of my head, had been cut out and sent halfway across the country. I was so focused on getting better that I hadn't taken the time to think about what actually had happened to me physically during surgery.

It was a great day, and I stopped myself from going down that dark path of worry. I got this! I thought instead as we all got in the car. Then, we teared up. We'd had amazing news.

I looked at my parents. All I could say was, "Thank you from the bottom of my heart. You guys know how much I love to be challenged, but this one was definitely has been rough. I couldn't have done this without you guys. Thank you for being such an phenomenal support system," I said, tears in my eyes,

It had been an incredible day, already, but there was one more thing I wanted to do. I asked my parents if we could stop at my house quickly.

I was uneasy about seeing where this calamity had struck me. Would I get flashbacks of the event? Would I pass out? I wanted to go there with people I trusted and felt safe with.

My parents did not hesitate. "Let's go," Dad said as he started to drive towards my house.

My heart was in my throat. It had been so long that I was confused about where I was. We pulled into my driveway. I had worked so hard to get to that point. My parents helped me out of the car. I was getting very good at doing things on my own, but my parents will always be parents, so they were concerned. That's what made them who they are. If I were 50, I'd still be their little boy.

I walked into the garage and up the two steps into my house, Dad behind me in case I lost my balance. I could smell the faint smell of fresh cotton air fresheners that I'd put around my house when I moved in.

I took a deep breath as I walked around the first floor. "I never thought I'd be back here," I said as I looked around. I was nervous to go up to the second floor, which is where I was when everything happened. I asked my parents if they were ready to go up there with me.

I proceeded slowly, step by step. I breathed deeply as I got closer to my room. I slowly looked around. I felt fine. Then I walked into the bathroom, the last place I remembered being before I woke up in the hospital. It was hard to believe all that had happened. The fact that my house was so close to the hospital was a major reason that I was alive.

"Okay, guys, I think I'm ready." I was smiling, and I could tell they wondered why I was so happy. "Well, I just accomplished another of my milestone goals."

I had figured out that setting small goals was the only way I would make it through, and that's exactly what seeing my house was. Content, I headed back to Kessler.

(ERICA)

ONCE I FOUND out what Dr. C had said, I was relieved. Joe was ahead of schedule, and that meant he had more time to recover. I saw that everything would click back into place much more quickly than we had anticipated. That was great. I was just very impatient and wanted everything to be better *now*. I knew that my initial reaction had been based on emotion. Getting factual information from the doctor made me feel much better.

I was also relieved that I had gone back to clean Joe's house after the paramedics had taken him to the hospital. For, as difficult as that had been for me, I knew I had to clean it up before anyone entered that house again. There was no point in keeping the scene as it was for everyone else to see. I had been able to prevent my parents from seeing that messy bathroom because I didn't want their imaginations to wander. It wasn't worth the pain.

Was it difficult for me to go back there so soon after? Hell, yeah! I'll never forget any of the events of that day. I'll forever remember what was said, what was done, who was there, and so on. But after some time, I realized that although that day had been hell, if anything had been different, my brother might not be alive today. I know this may sound weird, but I'm grateful for that day, grateful that God's plan was for Joe to be saved.

You don't know what you have in life until it's almost taken from you. I wanted to protect my entire family. Everyone was sad, Joe was hurt, and my parents were confused. What could I do to make it better for them? All I had to offer were my attention and time. My parents didn't need to *see* what had taken place in Joe's house that day. Nobody should have to see someone they love in a position like that. I just hoped that Joe's successful recovery would create new memories to take over this negative one. Wishful thinking, but this is what I prayed for every day.

LAST WEEKEND AT KESSLER (JOE AND ERICA)

(JOE)

MY LAST WEEKEND as an inpatient at Kessler was bittersweet. I owe so much to everyone I worked with and encountered at Kessler. Everyone pushed me hard and encouraged me to follow the process, and I made good progress during my recovery. But it was July 20, 2013, and Erica's twenty-ninth birthday, and I put my recovery on hold for the night.

I felt horrible that Erica had to celebrate her last birthday in her twenties at a rehabilitation hospital with me. I wished there was something I could do to give back the time to everyone who had to celebrate their birthdays in the rehab day room. I had a lot of making up to do, and I was determined to make it up to them in time.

The whole family was there to celebrate. We ordered a bunch of pizzas and joked and laughed and shared stories all evening. We invited some of the staff to come by for pizza if they could. We celebrated until late at night. I was exhausted but fought hard to stay awake. I love being around people, but I had begun to notice that I got over-stimulated when a lot was going on, and I tired extremely quickly. It was starting to annoy me. I *love* socializing. My family knows me so well that they notice immediately when I'm getting tired and call me out on it.

I woke up early on Sunday. My last couple of days would be busy as I went to any remaining appointments and therapy sessions. My parents and Erica helped me get my stuff together. I hadn't realized how many people had visited me, and more than I had realized had been kind enough to bring me gifts to lift my spirits. I needed a big suitcase to take it all home. There were balloons in the corner of my room and cases of sports drinks.

I took some time to reflect on the month I had been there. I have been associated with some wonderful people in my life, and I am grateful for it.

(ERICA)

I COULD TELL by Joe's face that he was unsure whether I was comfortable celebrating my birthday at Kessler. What he didn't understand was that I would never want to celebrate my birthday without him. Yeah, some friends wanted to take me to dinner to celebrate, so I made some plans for the other times that week, but I wanted to spend my actual birthday surrounded by my family.

Although that last weekend was tough since I wasn't ready for Joe to leave, we all enjoyed each other in that day room at Kessler. The entire wall was a window with a nice view. No matter what, the room was always bright. At night, you could see the lights of the entire town from that room. I will never forget that evening for as long as I live. My family was together, and we genuinely enjoyed ourselves. It wasn't about gifts or food. It was about the company. We joked around about old times. My brother made fun of me for getting old! My cousins were there laughing with us. If I'd been wearing a blindfold and couldn't have seen Joe in his wheelchair, I would have thought we were out to dinner—as we no doubt would have been on an average birthday. It was a comforting feeling. Joe would zone off when he was tired, and although I wanted to spend as much time with him as I could, I knew that he needed his rest in order to recover.

I missed seeing Joe at home in our familiar and comforting environment, but I had wanted him to be 100 percent back to himself before leaving. Even so, I was thrilled that soon I'd have my partner in crime back. That summer was one of the loneliest of my life. I had pushed many people away. Worst of all, I couldn't call my brother up and ask him to come to the diner or to see a movie. My best friend had been stuck in a rehab hospital, fighting for his strength.

Every time my mind wandered in a negative direction, I reminded myself how lucky I was that he was alive and progressing so well. Growing up, many people had poked fun at us because my parents had raised my brother and me to be close. I am grateful that they did, because it means my forever-best friend has always been in my family.

THAT'S A WRAP
(JOE AND ERICA)

(JOE)

ON MY NEXT to last day as an inpatient at Kessler, I was up early for my last therapy session. My occupational therapist, Kristen, came into my room to go over instructions for folding clothes, making the bed, and showering. She asked me to make the bed, fold the down comforter I had used during my stay, and put it in the closet. I hate folding clothes. I rolled the comforter up in a ball and shoved it into the closet.

"You're kidding me, right?" Kristen said.

I laughed. "What's the problem? Out of sight, out of mind, right?"

"You're a pain in the ass."

I took that as a compliment.

Then she made sure that I could give myself an unassisted shower. Given that the shower is the easiest place for someone to fall, she told me to use a shower chair. It was quite a process, but I was glad to shower on my own again. Being twenty-seven and having to rely on other people to assist me in the shower would have stripped away any dignity I might have had left after all I'd been through.

We walked down to the outpatient gym on the first floor to meet my outpatient physical therapist, Tyler. I couldn't wait to get back into therapy. I had many goals to achieve and didn't want to waste any time. Wanting to do something nice for all of the doctors and therapists, my parents brought a tray of assorted wraps and put them in the day room for the staff to enjoy. It was the least we could do to repay them for all they had done for my family and me.

After lunch, we finished my final paperwork and made sure that everything from my room was accounted for. The next morning, I would leave Kessler early. I was happy to take that next step towards normalcy, but I knew that I would miss the constant push for a faster recovery. My doctors and therapists were no longer just doctors and therapists to me. I consider every one of them a friend, and I made it a point to visit as often as possible

It wouldn't have been normal for us to quietly leave Kessler without a last night of celebration, and we did just that. We had one last big, Italian family dinner at Kessler, laughing noisily, eating, and swapping stories with the staff and each other.

This was it. I had done it. I had recovered to the point where I could go home! After my family went home and I was back in my room by myself, left to reminisce. I could hardly believe what I had accomplished.

On June 9, 2013, I had lost movement and feeling on the left side of my body. A surgeon cut a hole on the right side of my head to drain the fluid and eliminate any pressure caused by the bleed, and it was expected that I would have a *long* recovery. No one wanted me to know all the negative things they had been told about my condition. I can't be mad at the doctors for making my family aware of the possibilities. Even if there had been just the slightest possibility that something would happen, they needed to say it: *He might never walk, talk, see, or regain any movement on his left side.* I discovered my limitations during my recovery, and I used the information as motivation.

I said then, and I still say, "Tell me something I can't do, and I will prove you wrong." I love a good challenge. There I was, lying in bed on my last night as an inpatient only two months or so after my AVM had ruptured. I was walking, talking, joking, and most important, I was positive and ready to defy the odds.

(ERICA)

GETTING READY FOR Joe's arrival was both exciting and nerve racking. My mom cleaned our house from top to bottom, got brand-new towels, and in every way made sure that the house was up to par for Joe. I put together his shower chair, checking it twenty times to make sure I had done it correctly. We wanted Joe to be comfortable and to have everything he needed.

I could barely contain myself. I got some movies and thought about what we could do to keep busy. Joe would be wearing his helmet, so we would have to be careful about his movements. I was so happy that he would be in a familiar, comfortable place. There would be no more shots and no more nurses and doctors around. It would be just family and friends, and that's exactly how I liked it. My brother was coming back!

My new house would have to take a back seat. My family needed me and, to be honest, I needed them. All of us had to work together for Joe. We wanted to make sure that he stayed in good spirits and was never alone. We had almost lost him once, and we were going to make sure that he was safe and with his loved ones.

I hoped that he wasn't worried about being alone. However, one thing I had learned during this experience was that I had more fears in my heart and mind than Joe could ever think of. I wondered whether this was a personality trait I'd always had, or whether Joe's trauma had triggered a new fear. I realized I was developing a chronic state of anxiety. It wasn't fun, but it seemed to keep me on my toes in dealing with Joe's recovery.

I hoped that it would go away once he was recovered.

HOME! (JOE AND ERICA)

(JOE)

AT SIX A.M. on July 23, 2013, the nursing staff woke me up. I was exhausted. It took me a while to realize what was going on. When my dad came in with my usual breakfast, it hit me.

"Up and at 'em! I'm ready to take my boy home."

I could see how happy he was just by the look in his eyes. My dad had been my wingman and my buddy every step of the way. When I hear people say parents can't be friends with their kids, I think that is an absolute lie. My father is like a brother and friend to me. I respect him for everything he has done and sacrificed for my family and me. He never complained about a thing. It's him I strive to be like when I get married and become a father.

What was killing me inside about my situation was what would happen if I didn't achieve my goals. Would I ever be able to take care of kids and a wife as I had watched my father do for all these years?

Throughout my journey, I spoke with my dad about this plenty of times. He uttered his infamous word, the one he said whenever I had any doubts: "Yet." He unfailingly reassured me that, with patience and hard work, things would work out.

That day was a bit different, though. I didn't have to be patient. I was going home!

My mom had the house all set up for me. She had bought new, white towels for me when I showered to ensure I didn't get any infections. My parents also had sacrificed their bed for me because they knew how uncomfortable I was sleeping with a hole in my head. I begged them not to, to take it back, but there was no way I would win that fight, so eventually I gave up.

After I walked around the house for a few minutes, taking it all in, I was beat. I lay down on the bed to just relax and think for a couple of minutes, and four hours later, I woke up. That nap felt wonderful! I had waited so long to feel comfortable in bed.

"I have a question for you," I said to my mom. "So, how does this work? Do I get a bell or something for when I need you to help me with something?" I grinned at her.

She laughed. "I'll give you a bell!"

It felt good to be home. The same as it was when I was still in the hospital; friends and family came by to visit. I received text message after text message welcoming me home. It felt good to be loved. I wish that everyone at some point in life could feel the love that I had felt over those months. I swore I would give back and make someone else feel on top of the world someday. That had become my ultimate goal. I would not consider myself recovered until I was making a difference for others.

(ERICA)

ONE OF THE most emotional parts of the ordeal had been watching Joe sleep. I could tell how uncomfortable he was. He had to sleep on one side all the time, and because he's so tall, the beds in the hospital and in rehab were never long enough for him. It bothered me that he couldn't at least be in the comfort of his own bed. On his first day home, I went upstairs to say hi to him, but he was sleeping. I felt immediately comforted. I was happy to see him in his familiar environment, his legs not hanging over the edge of a bed, and his helmet tucked to the side of him. Joe was able to take his helmet off when he slept, even though it scared the hell out of me. I watched him for over an hour.

I was emotional for many reasons: sad that this had happened to him and angry that he had to wear a helmet because he was missing part of his skull. I was happy that he was home with our family. So many thoughts were tumbling through my head that I couldn't contain myself. I had been strong in front of him since the rupture, but that day I couldn't contain myself. I kept crying, probably to let out feelings I had repressed.

I had to get myself together and stop thinking about my sadness. I looked in the mirror, and then splashed cold water on my face. I looked different—older and not my usual happy self.

Would I ever be the same again? Would my sadness go away? I wanted life to go back to normal. Every night I fell asleep, hoping that when I woke up, I'd realize I'd had a nightmare and it was over. But each morning I'd wake up and have to relive the entire situation through memories all over again.

OUTPATIENT BEGINS
(JOE AND ERICA)

(JOE)

MY FIRST DAY of outpatient therapy with Tyler was fairly simple. We got to know each other and came to an understanding about my goals for recovery. I spoke of my desire to play basketball again. A league started in the fall. I wanted to get my recovery over with and play in a pickup game of basketball. He did a balance test so we'd have a starting point for measuring my improvement. I understood the difference between inpatient and outpatient right away. When I was an inpatient, the goal seemed to be getting me to a point where I could go home. Outpatient therapy placed greater focus on my longer-term goals. I was pumped and ready for that challenge, ready to work hard.

The next day, I had to reschedule therapy to go to an appointment with a neuro-ophthalmologist, who wasn't affiliated with Kessler. He would test my visual field and fix it, and I'd finally be back to normal.

I just knew everything would turn out great. Nothing could bring me down because the worst was behind me. I'd endured extreme physical pain and intense emotional and mental challenges. I'd learned to walk again and was able to use my left side fully. It's not common having to face those challenges out of nowhere. This visual challenge might be my last. I couldn't wait to see the world like I used to. I'd never take anything for granted again.

(ERICA)

AT FIRST, I had worried that Joe wouldn't be given any more therapy once he was out of rehab. Since I'd found out that he'd still get therapy, I was excited for him. He still had room for improvement, and he was going to make it. Joe had impressed me greatly in how he'd dealt with his ordeal. Before the rupture, happened, Joe had had a tendency to give up on things when they became too difficult for him, and I'd been afraid that he'd give up and not work very hard. He proved me wrong. He was up and ready to go to therapy hours before he had to leave. I was surprised at his focus on his goals. I just knew that he would meet them all.

I went shopping. I wanted to get Joe something to signify the beginning of his life outside of the hospital. It had to be something good. At last, I found the perfect gift: sneakers! They were red-and-black basketball sneakers that he could wear to his therapy sessions. That day, price didn't matter. I couldn't wait to see the delight on his face. I also got him sweatpants, a few pairs of shorts, and some t-shirts. He was all set. I wanted him to be comfortable during his therapy sessions. Not to mention, these were things that he had enjoyed before his rupture. Purchasing these items brought me back to a sort of familiarity and sense of comfort.

BUMP IN THE ROAD
(JOE AND ERICA)

(JOE)

TO ME, MY vision was the final issue. With time and hard work, I knew I'd get back to jogging and regain my strength, but there was absolutely nothing I could do about my vision on my own. I was left with hopes and dreams that one day I'd wake up and see the world as I used to.

I heard my name called. It was time. My parents and I went into the exam room. I took a bunch of tests in which I had to click every time I saw a light. It was not easy. The assistant took the results to the doctor and led us into another room. I was nervous about what was to come.

I talked with my parents. "I have a good feeling about how I did. I'm hoping they'll tell me there's medicine or contacts or something that will make everything go back to normal."

Noticing that I was nervous, Dad picked up a little skeleton head next to him and fiddled around with it. We all laughed hysterically. He put the skeleton head down just in time. The doctor came in.

Well, it was time.

"Hi, Joe," he said. "I took a look at the results and studied the images that were taken for some time. Do you want the good news or the bad news, first?" His tone was serious.

My heart was beating fast, and I felt sick to my stomach. "Just give me the bad news. I mean, how bad can it be?"

"You have hemianopsia in both eyes, and most likely your normal vision won't come back. The good news is that you still have half your vision, and there are some things that can help you function a little better with what you have."

I didn't understand what he meant by that. Hemianopsia? I just stared at him. What was that? There had to be something to fix it. I mean, the way he'd said it meant there had to be something to follow that up. I said, "What does hemianopsia mean?" I felt dumb.

"You lost half of your visual field to the left in both eyes. So, if you draw a vertical line straight down the center of both eyes, you only see what is to the right. It means half-blind in both eyes."

My face felt white, like all the blood had drained out of it. I felt my heart in my throat. My eyes filled up. I looked up at my parents. They were stunned and had no words to comfort me. I asked for options to make this better.

He gave me some glasses to try on and told me to walk back and forth down the hall. This told me nothing except that they didn't work.

When we went to the desk, I dared to ask him about driving.

"Joe, you have lost half of your vision. If you were my son, I'd say you're never going to drive again. Look into other means of transportation." He said this snappishly, as if he were smacking me for asking such a stupid question.

That was when I felt my world come crashing down on me. It felt like a movie in slow motion. I felt my legs giving out and got so nauseated that I thought I was going to vomit. My parents grabbed a chair and put it behind me. I fell into it. I tried to take deep breaths. Nothing was working.

"Okay, let's go," I said to my parents.

I don't know if I said another word to the doctor. I remember that my dad talked to him for a minute or two, but I was still reeling and didn't remember another thing that had happened in that office. I got into the passenger seat, and my mom and dad got in. It was silent for a good 30 seconds. My dad was trying to say something, but I heard nothing. I was a mess. Tears rolled down my face. Someone had just turned my life upside down. There was no positive end in sight.

I started to yell. "What did I ever do to God to make him do this to me? Who did I hurt? What did I ever do? I'm sorry! This can't be right! There's no way this guy is telling us the truth. Why is he such an asshole? He didn't even care! Did you see how heartless he was? Why?" I yelled and yelled. I was in a fog. I couldn't believe what that doctor had said to me.

My parents tried to say and do whatever they could to make me feel better. Nothing worked. I was beyond depressed. I wanted to be left alone. There was nothing left to live for. I was screwed. I could never be a father to any kids in my state. I couldn't even drive them to school if I wanted to. How was I going to get to work? I couldn't take it anymore.

I was silent as Dad drove us to Erica's house. She was grilling. I went inside and sat on the couch, emotionless and silent. I couldn't explain what had happened. I just sat there in silence. The rest of the day was a blur. I wanted to sleep and never wake up again. Maybe this was just a dream....

(ERICA)

THE DAY STARTED off great. My brother and my parents were coming over for a barbecue, and I had invited some friends. It was the first get–together at my house since my brother's initial surgery. I bought too much food.

I was optimistic that Joe's appointment would go well. At Kessler, they had mentioned that potentially his vision could come back. His sensation was slowly improving and he was walking more easily. His vision was probably next.

Then my parents called me. I could tell by their voices that the appointment had not gone as planned. I listened to them for a while. They told me the bad news, and all I could do was picture my brother's reaction.

I hung up the phone, put my head in my hands, and cried. What more could Joe go through? What else had to happen to him? I didn't understand why God was doing all these things to my brother. He'd always been such a good-hearted guy. Why couldn't he catch a break? I had guests, but I couldn't bring myself to go back outside. I needed to catch my breath.

When my parents and Joe arrived, I could tell that Joe was trying to be polite. After a bit, though, he went inside and sat on the couch, looking really depressed. When I asked, he told me what had happened: His vision would not be returning. He would never drive again. Despite the fact that he had been so positive, this news was a blow.

I wondered how he was going to deal with it. I started thinking about what we could do to help him. How much would a personal driver cost? Would the state pay for a program that could help him get places? Would he be able to keep his job?

It was all too much at once, and I wanted to fix all of it.

My brother's life had been changed drastically. I had been waiting for every change to be fixed, and he would go back to his old self. This news was a dose of reality; it told me that maybe life as Joe had known it wouldn't be exactly the same now.

As a counselor, I knew that people lived through losses throughout their lives. Life throws curve balls every day. When you go through tough changes, you have to make adjustments and work through the changes. Well, I wasn't ready to process or accept any of this. I wanted to avoid this nightmare.

The worst part was that I couldn't make him feel better. I had no words. Nothing would work. He was a mess, and there was nothing I could say or do to make it all stop. Helpless and out of options, all I could do was listen and let him cry. He had to process the loss of his vision for himself before he would be able to put the pieces back together and move forward. It was going to suck.

DIGESTING THE NEWS
(JOE AND ERICA)

(JOE)

I'D BE LYING if I said I took the news well. I didn't. I had an extremely hard time with it. It would affect every aspect of my life.

The next several weeks were rough. The news I'd received was emotionally devastating. I went to outpatient therapy several mornings a week, but I was disheartened. At night, I distracted myself with music, movies, and sports. While watching TV, every once in a while, I felt an emptiness in the pit of my stomach: What if I never got to see the world the way I used to? I'd never be able to play competitive sports again. Every time those thoughts came, I felt like I might vomit.

"Come on, Joe," I urged myself. "You can't think like that. You're alive. Remember, you can achieve anything that you put your mind to."

I literally tried anything I could to distract myself from my reality. Reflecting back, it probably wasn't the best way to approach the situation. I didn't talk out my feelings with someone so I could come to terms with them. I felt bad every time I mentioned anything to my parents or sister. It wasn't fair, because they couldn't do anything to fix it. I was miserable, but why should I make them miserable, too?

One day, something clicked. I could not allow myself to stay in that rut. People looked up to me for what I had accomplished so far. I couldn't let my little cousins down. They admired me. My family had been my rock since day one, and I'd be letting them down, too.

That's it, I thought. Enough feeling bad for myself. I *needed* to get my life back on track. It was time to man up and go at my recovery headfirst.

I got up ready to work hard. I lifted light weights, even though I wasn't supposed to. It was a way to let out my anger and frustrations. I got up the next morning for outpatient therapy. I worked hard, praying every day that my vision would randomly come back and I'd prove that asshole of a doctor wrong. My therapist, Tyler, would laugh and throw me a towel the moment I came in because I always sweated profusely. I constantly pushed myself as hard as I could.

Time flew by, and my progress skyrocketed. Soon, I was cleared to get up and walk around the house without assistance. Finally, I felt free. I didn't have to wait for someone to follow me to the bathroom to make sure I was okay.

On August 16, 2013, my family took me down the shore for the first time since the rupture. It was exciting to be outside, walking around again. Every day I got up with the family, and we walked on the boardwalk for hours. We laughed because when I took my helmet off, I had a helmet tan. If you can't make yourself laugh, you're not living.

It was just the trip I needed to clear my mind and enjoy a little vacation from reality. When I got back home, I continued to work hard to defy the odds.

(ERICA)

THE WEEKS THAT followed Joe's appointment with the neuro-opthalmologist were terrible. Joe changed. He wasn't the same as he'd been in the hospital and rehab hospital. He was down and couldn't pick himself up. He was still having difficulty processing the loss of half of his vision. Again, I ignored the fact that I had to accept these changes in my brother; instead, I spent every day trying to make him smile. It felt like I trying to run through a brick wall. I was relentless, but no matter how fast I ran, I fell on my face. Each time, I'd get a new bruise, but I'd get up and try again. It was an impossible task, and I was completely worn out.

The family came up with the idea of going down the shore to try to enjoy what was left of the summer. I didn't expect Joe to agree to come along. But then his attitude changed, and he wanted to try something new. I didn't understand completely; Joe's internal dialogue was personal to him. He was the only one who could sort through his emotions and feelings. Nobody could do that for him. But whatever he was thinking, he was still taking steps forward, and that was the best news in the world.

The time at the shore was heartwarming. Joe was active and ready to be around us all. Generally, I found it difficult to go back to the old places we'd been before his brain injury. I'd remember old times together and how awesome they were. This time, Joe was wearing a helmet. Looking at him, I'd catch myself reminiscing and getting sad. But every time, I told myself to stop and be thankful that he was alive. I needed to accept these changes, but I wasn't ready to do that. Unfortunately, this would become a problem later down the line.

FOLLOWING MY PASSION (JOE AND ERICA)

(JOE)

OVER THE NEXT several weeks after we returned from our trip down the shore, I realized that I needed to start doing things that made me happy.

Ever since I was really little, I've loved sports. I collected cards and autographed memorabilia. After receiving the phone call from John Starks, the video from Tiki Barber, and an autographed Derrick Rose jersey from my buddy Chris, I was ready to resume my childhood hobby. I couldn't play the sports I wanted to, but I could do what I could to follow my passion and to meet those athletes and thank them for helping me survive a difficult time. I was instantly drawn back into it. I did hours of research to catch up on the advances in the memorabilia industry: the latest on which pens to use on various objects, the best ways to preserve items, and the best items to get a signature on. I looked up all the signings in my area.

I considered going to signings part of my rehabilitation. I went to outpatient therapy a few days a week. On my days off, I worked out in the morning and did all of my home exercises. After Mom got home from work, we went to the signings. On the weekends, I went with Dad or Erica.

I had the opportunity to meet some inspirational athletes. A few stood out for me.

When I met Jason Pierre-Paul of the New York Giants, he saw me in my helmet and asked if I was okay. We talked for a couple of minutes. I explained what had happened, and he said something similar had happened to one of his former teammates. Just the fact that he let others wait and talked to me for a little while to make sure I was okay showed the type of individual he is.

The athlete who impressed me the most was by far Mike Tyson. I went into Brooklyn to his book signing. Lots of people were there. I waited for some time, standing there with my book open to the page I wanted him to sign. Finally, it was my turn. Mike Tyson! It was so cool.

I went up to the table where he sitting. "Champ, I have two questions for you." I smiled, while security was instructing me to follow the process quickly. He signed my book.

"When are you going to come out of retirement? Because I can't deal with how boring the heavyweight division has gotten."

He laughed heartily.

"Which hurts worse—a knockout punch by you in your prime or this?" I appointed to my incision. My incision was still pretty raw at the time, and my head was still shaved from my surgeries. I turned my head to the side for him to see.

"Come over here by me," he said, making the other fans wait. "What happened?"

I explained my situation and what I had overcome during the last several months.

"What have the doctors said? Did they say you were going to be okay?" he asked in a concerned voice as he shook my hand.

I looked him right in the eyes and said, "Champ, I know you've been told plenty of times that you couldn't do something and you did it. I don't care what anyone tells me about whether or not I'm going to be okay. I pave my own path in life, and I decide whether or not I'll be okay."

He glanced at the security guards and leaned closer to me. I will never forget his next words. "Listen, I'm not the real champ. I'm talking to the real champ."

I was astonished to hear that from one of the best boxers ever.

He turned to the security people and said, "Do you believe this guy?" To me, he said, "Thank you for sharing your story with me. Don't give up. Keep on fighting."

"Did that really just happen?" I thought. I couldn't stop talking about it for days.

I knew what I wanted to do next. I had an empty room at my house. It was time for me to display my collection. I would turn my spare room into an office/sport memorabilia room. I couldn't wait!

(ERICA)

EVERY TIME WE met a new athlete, I got emotional. I never knew how strangers would react to my brother. Being a protective sister, I worried that they would disappoint him. But I have to say that every athlete he met was receptive and friendly. Hearing Joe's stories about the words these people used to empathize and encourage was touching. Meeting these sports figures made my brother happy. They were genuinely impressed with his progress. They hadn't known him before, but they knew him now. After all Joe had gone through, he was still being able to motivate and impress others. I was and I am lucky to be Joe's sister. These athletes inspired Joe, and they were even more inspired by him. I couldn't have been prouder.

I had always been skeptical of people and their intentions, but Joe was a like a magnet. People flocked to him. His smile was contagious. People wanted to hear his story and learn more about him.

My anxiety about others' reactions to him dissipated a bit more with each new encounter. Joe is great, and everyone who meets him knows it. Joe wasn't meeting celebrities; they were meeting him, and they loved him.

CLOSE ME UP! (JOE AND ERICA)

(JOE)

THE REST OF the summer went by quickly. I worked hard every day. I spent a lot of time getting my typing going again. I spent a lot of time reading to train my eyes to continue looking to the left. I made everything I did as difficult as possible so I could train myself to be that much better. I continued to follow up with my doctors at Kessler, who said I was progressing very well.

Football season came on in full force. That was exciting; it was a way for me to socialize and be around people. Crowds were tough to navigate with only half my vision in both eyes, and I looked at it as a challenge. With every great challenge comes great reward. I had faith that this challenge would improve my condition.

Thanksgiving came. I was extremely thankful that year. I was alive, and to be quite honest, I'm not sure how. I felt I was kept alive for a reason. I determined that I would figure out what that reason was and do something big with it. I would give back to those in need.

Just as fast as Thanksgiving came, it went. On December 1, 2013, I had my final surgery. Doctors put the bone flap back into my head and closed me up. The night before, I looked forward to it, relieved that I would finally get out of that helmet. I had spent almost six months wearing a bike helmet.

I was also nervous. What would happen if they put my bone in and my brain swelled and hit my skull? What if I didn't look the same anymore? What if I woke up immobile again? I sure didn't want to go through the same thing again. I had no clue what to expect.

Starting at midnight, I wasn't allowed to eat or drink anything. Up until then, I made sure to drink one or two glasses of water an hour. It was not fun to think about the operation. I had to be at the hospital by seven a.m., and before then, I had to take an antibacterial shower to ensure that I was as free as possible of any bacteria. I listened to music and thought that at this time the next day, I'd be out of the helmet and back together. I packed my bag for the hospital stay, including stuff to do while lying in bed. I fell asleep as I was thinking and trying to relax.

The alarm on the morning of my surgery seemed to go off just minutes after I had fallen asleep.

"Here we go!" I said as I woke up. I was going out in public with that awful helmet for the last time.

Dad made coffee for him and Mom. The aroma was killing me since I couldn't drink any. I was very tired, but my nerves and excitement kept me going.

After we had sat for a while in the waiting room, my name was called. I went through the paperwork routine. One question had always puzzled: what pain level don't you ever want to get above, on a scale of 0 to 10. I question the intelligence of anyone who answers anything other than 0.

I was all set and ready for Dr. C to come in before they rolled me into the operating room. My parents and Erica were with me, and we were all smiling and laughing. That was how we coped when we were nervous—or at least how I did.

And then it was time. The anesthesiologist came in. Just as he was about to administer the anesthesia, I said, "I'll see you guys with a full skull! I love you! Hey, wait—I got this!" I said, holding my fist up in the air.

I woke up in a lot of pain. Feeling staples holding your scalp together is not fun. Five titanium plates with five screws in each plate held my bone in place.

"Damn, that's pretty badass," I thought.

My head was completely bandaged, and there was a drain in my scalp so no excess fluid could build up. They wheeled me to the step down unit where they administered more medication and let me recover.

It was December 3, 2013. Dr. C came in to check in on me. "It's pretty badass to have all those plates and screws, so I wanted to round out the look for you."

He took off the bandages, and there it was—a Mohawk. I laughed and figured why the hell not.

It was time for the drain to come out. The nurse put one hand on my head and gave the tube a yank. Pop! It came out. This was followed by a clicking sound and a sharp pain at the top of my head. My dad cringed as he watched. I could have done without feeling my head get stapled, but by then, I was so numb to the pain that it barely fazed me. I was elated to be done. Two weeks later, all of the staples were removed, and I was ready to get on with my life.

(ERICA)

THANKSGIVING WAS THE worst. On the following Monday, Joe would have surgery. Thanksgiving was the first big holiday we'd all spent together after Joe's third surgery. During those few months, I felt like things were kind of back together. I was accustomed to having Joe home, and I loved it. From the moment I walked into my aunt's house on Thanksgiving, I felt sick to my stomach. Every year we took a Thanksgiving photo with my cousins and my grandmother in front of the turkey. I kept thinking of Joe having to be in the photo with his helmet on.

My family noticed that I was getting overwhelmed that night. I didn't want to get emotional in front of my brother, so I left the room so I could let out my emotions. I sat with my aunt for a while. I cried and asked her how she had gotten the images from the very first day out of her head. She had been with me when we got to Joe's house, she was with me in the ER that day, and she saw exactly what I saw. My nightmares never stopped. I often woke up in the middle of the night, sweating, from dreaming that I didn't make it to Joe on time. Other nights, I dreamed that I didn't tell Joe to call 911 that day. It was horrible, and for some reason, on that Thanksgiving night, it all got to me.

My aunt told me she couldn't stop thinking of that day, either. She, too, was having nightmares. She cried with me. "It's so difficult, but we have to move on from it for Joe's sake."

I tried my best. I knew that it was necessary. But it was so much easier said than done. That traumatic day was catching up with me. I had avoided the thoughts for so long, but I couldn't forget the memory. Flashbacks came and took me over. I had talked to my brother while his brain was bleeding. I had seen the paramedics lift him out. I talked to him while he was in the emergency room, slowly losing consciousness. All these scenes had taken over my mind, and by Thanksgiving, I'd had enough. I felt guilty if I talked to my parents about that day. They didn't know the details, and they didn't need to know. I didn't confide in friends. I just wanted to avoid it all, but I couldn't. The memories had become my worst enemy. I had been running from them, but I was losing energy. The thoughts and images had unlimited energy, and by then they were outrunning me.

When Joe had to go in for his surgery, I was petrified. I didn't think I could take another waiting game. I sat there and watched him go through the routine: changing into his hospital gown, getting hooked up to machines. Doctors and nurses walked in and out of the area where he was waiting. Every time I felt my eyes filling up, I'd put my head down. I couldn't let Joe see me cry. This had become far too familiar; I just wanted to move forward. This would be it, I knew. He'd finally be done with all of the crap. I doubt I could have been more nervous and happy at the same time.

BOSCO (JOE AND ERICA)

(JOE)

SOON, I WAS back in outpatient therapy at Kessler. Therapy was much easier without a helmet. The scabbing was falling off, and I was back in business. I made incredible progress. I was not as nervous about falling once I had the bone flap back in my head. Before, I hadn't been able to do any jumping or running because it gave me a killer headache. My brain was pressurizing, so I was able to gradually increase the intensity of my exercise. My confidence was building.

I kept thinking back to when I was an inpatient and how different I had been then. I spent a lot of time reflecting. I kept remembering the moment I fell when I was walking the dog in inpatient and about the therapy dogs that had visited me in the hospital. I had felt defeated and was trying to make up for it by challenging myself. I wanted a dog of my own. Some people tried to tell me that I was in no position to get a dog, that there was no way I could handle that responsibility. Their discouragement only made me more determined.

I spoke with my family about my idea. I weighed it all out. Having a dog would push me to get up and walk every day. A dog would make me chase after him.

The right dog for me, I decided, was an English Bulldog. I saw a picture online of my perfect dog, and I knew I had to have him. I arranged to get my puppy on January 24, 2014. We all sat around the living room discussing the ideal name for my new buddy, throwing out names like Tyson, Brutus, and Capone. And then Erica said it—Bosco. It would be perfect for my brindle-and-white English Bulldog.

I couldn't wait to pick up Bosco. I researched and made sure I had everything ready for him. I had loads of toys and all. My house was completely puppy-proofed. I was reading books on training. I couldn't get enough. Bit by bit, I began moving stuff back into my new house and staying there from time to time. At first, my dad stayed with me, then my sister, and sometimes I stayed on my own to boost my confidence about being alone.

That Christmas in 2013 was extra meaningful. I had so much to say to my family that I had no clue where to begin. Everyone had been there for me through the whole ordeal. I was extremely emotional at Christmas time. I shouldn't have been there, but I was. That's all I kept thinking and saying to everyone. "Thank you" were the words that kept coming out of my mouth.

Christmas seemed to pass in the blink of an eye. On New Year's Eve, I celebrated because 2013 was coming to an end. No more surgeries and nothing but happy, healthy, and positive thoughts.

(ERICA)

JOE WANTED A dog. Good idea? I didn't know about that! He was still recovering, and I sure as hell didn't know anything about animals. We didn't grow up with a dog in the house, so I really couldn't be of much help to him.

One night, he showed me a picture online of the cutest English Bulldog I had ever seen. The name he had already been given was Bear. After looking at him for a while, I knew that he had to be named Bosco. I even liked Bosco Bear. I didn't know what was going to happen, but I knew that I would learn, because this dog wasn't even there yet but he was already making Joe happy.

We looked at the website for hours. Every time I asked Joe if he wanted to watch a movie, he ignored my question and showed me another picture of the puppy. For Joe, it was love at first sight, so that dog had to be his. My mom was worried about him taking care of a new puppy, but Joe was determined. One thing that had not changed about Joe was that, once he had his heart and mind set on something, it had to happen.

I did more research on the therapeutic benefits of pets. Maybe a dog would be good for him. I was worried and excited at the same time.

BACK TO REALITY
(JOE AND ERICA)

(JOE)

ON JANUARY 14, 2014, I had to tackle another challenge. After more than half a year and four surgeries, I headed back to work at my job in the business world.

As I was going through my recovery, I heard that some people had said I'd need to be out far longer, and others had questioned whether I would ever be able to return to work. I said it once, and I continue to say it: Tell me more that I can't do so I can show you otherwise. I had worked extremely hard to get back on my feet, literally and metaphorically. I had challenged myself physically, mentally, and emotionally to get back to a normal life. I had a house to pay for, a future to save for, and people to inspire.

I was happy to go back to work and see everyone. Many of my colleagues had come to visit while I was at Overlook and Kessler. They had seen me at my worst. Everyone spoke about how much of a struggle I'd had and how difficult that was. The crazy thing is, I didn't quite understand it myself, yet.

My mom took me to work, and my dad picked me up. I hated adding this complexity to my family's lives. It sucked, to be quite honest. It was nothing I could control, but I wished that there was something I could do. I researched programs that potentially could give me a ride to and from work without burdening anyone. The more I thought about being a burden, the more upset I got. But I couldn't let it faze me. I needed to be at my best. I got up just as it began to get light, ready to go back to work and make my first appearance without a helmet.

I arrived at work and met with a colleague. A 2014 planning meeting took up the whole day. To be honest, when I heard about it, I had no idea how I would hold up. In the event, I did my best to contribute and listen. I was struggling, but I couldn't show it. After an hour or two, I was dead tired. What was going on? I'd just had two cups of coffee. I commanded myself to wake up. I don't know how, but I made it through the rest of the day.

When Dad picked me up after work, he took a look at me and asked what was wrong.

"I barely made it through the day. I don't know what's wrong with me! After an hour of just listening to conversations and trying to see who was talking, I'm completely exhausted."

"Maybe you didn't get enough sleep."

I didn't have an answer, but I was scared. I had never been so tired from doing nothing.

Time went on, and I continued to truck through. I struggled to keep my poker face on. I had never liked to show defeat, and I absolutely did not want to be defeated. Sometimes, when I couldn't handle the headaches and exhaustion, I'd go for a fifteen-minute walk or go into the bathroom to wash my face and be in silence for a few minutes. This went on for some time, and it sucked. I figured that the harder I tried to push through, the sooner it would get easier.

After a little over a week back at work, the big day came—the day I picked up Bosco. It was a remarkable distraction from my headaches. I loved him from the second I got him. He was a ten-pound bundle of joy. The first time I held him, he fell asleep in my arms and started snoring. I knew instantly that I had made the right decision. For the next couple of months, a coworker would take me back to my house at lunch to let Bosco out. On days that I couldn't get a ride during lunch, Mom or another family member let him out during lunch. Again, my family was always there for me when I needed them. I didn't realize it at the time, but the constant running around after Bosco and taking him outside for walks helped my coordination and walking ability immensely.

I decided to challenge myself even further. This probably won't come as a surprise, but I told my friends that I owed it to them to play kickball again. We had just started a league when my trouble struck, so I had missed the whole season. I decided I'd play kickball on a team with them. I knew I wasn't very good, but I found it thrilling to do even the slightest things, like making contact with the ball and not hitting the floor while trying. The first time I made it on base, my friends cheered and high-fived me and all that good stuff.

I can't even think of the words to describe how it made me feel. I did something I had promised them I'd do again. I went out on a whim and pushed myself to do it. I may have run like Frankenstein, but I didn't care because I was out there, and I was having fun with my friends. God is good!

(ERICA)

JOE'S FIRST DAY of work was an emotional one for us all. I had faith that he could do it, but again, I was afraid that if he had a difficult time, he'd give up. I was used to Joe feeling defeated at times before his brain injury. Although it seemed that he was much more confident and daring now, I still worried that he would quit things. I prayed that everything would run smoothly. I wanted him to be successful.

My parents and I took turns driving Joe to work. People asked me if it was out of our way to take Joe to work. I thought they must be morons. We had spent months in the hospital and rehab hospital. My brother had had to wear a helmet. Did I really give a crap that I had to drive an extra half hour out of my way to help him out? How could anyone in their right mind think that we would make him fend for himself? That was never an option.

I couldn't watch Joe play kickball again for the first time. I just couldn't watch. I feel horrible about this now, but I wasn't ready. I've always been a strong person. Even the nature of my profession involves helping students and families work through the most difficult times. But watching my brother potentially get disappointed or upset was not an option. I had to avoid it. I give my parents all the credit in the world; if they were worried about him getting upset or not being successful, they never showed it, not once. Their strength was endless. Meanwhile, my emotions got the better of me. When I heard that the kickball game went well and he'd had a great time, I was so happy. It was absolutely wonderful news.

And Bosco. Since he had arrived, Joe was a changed person. He made sure that dog was taken care of. I'll never forget the night Bosco arrived. I had slept over at Joe's house so we could take care of the dog. We were up pretty much every hour. I hadn't realized how much work a puppy could be. Joe had read books, watched videos, and done hours of research on how to take care of his new best friend. From the beginning, he was a great dad to that puppy.

UH-OH (JOE AND ERICA)

(JOE)

THE WINTER ENDED and the warmer weather arrived. It was May of 2014. I had been doing so well, but I was struggling at work. I was having such horrible headaches that I couldn't concentrate. They felt like dull, never-ending migraines. I was showing up at work and doing whatever I could to stay focused. I sat at my desk and sometimes just had to put my head in my hands and press on my temples. I had no clue what was causing the headaches, which had been going on for a few weeks.

Then, I looked in the mirror one morning and saw that there was an indentation on the right side of my head. I didn't remember seeing it before. Was that supposed to happen? Maybe the bone was growing and reattaching to my existing skull. I felt around the area and touched what I thought were the plates connecting the bone to my skull. That couldn't be good! I raised my eyebrows and heard a click. That was probably not a good sign, either.

I called my parents. "I think I feel the plates!" I shouted.

They tried to reassure me that everything was okay.

I really, really didn't think so. I went into work after the scare.

My dad called me. "I need you to go with your mom to the plastic surgeon's office. You have a one o'clock appointment."

I told my boss, who was cool with it and said to let him know what happened.

I figured nothing was going to be wrong. Maybe I would need a small adjustment, or maybe I thought I felt something that I didn't.

The doctor looked at my head and saw the indentation. He pressed on the indentation, and I felt a sharp pain in my head.

What the hell was going on?

The doctor took Mom and me into his office. I didn't know what he was going to say. My mom was sitting to my right. I was nervous.

The words he said next shocked the hell out of me. "I don't think your bone flap is there, anymore."

I'm sure my face turned white. "Excuse me?" I stared at him. "Well, I didn't take it out, so where the hell did it go?"

"You need to call Dr. C's office immediately and schedule an MRI."

"I don't understand. Where is my bone?" I was confused.

"It depends. You need to call Dr. C and find out if the bone is there or not. I can't tell for sure, but I don't think it is."

Either way, I was looking at another surgery, at the least. I called Dr. C's office and scheduled my MRI for that evening. I went back to work. I didn't have any words to say to anyone. I just went back for my things. I needed to take the rest of the day off. There was no way I'd be able to concentrate on anything else.

I went for an MRI, and I had an appointment with Dr. C a few days later. When Dad and I checked in, we saw Dr. C in the back office, squinting at the computer, with a serious look on his face. I glanced at my dad and knew he had noticed the doctor's expression. I felt flushed and clammy.

We seated ourselves in his office. Dr. C came in and shook our hands.

"Okay, so I took a look at the images," he said as he sat down. "I'm sorry, but it looks like there are only fragments of the bone left. I can see in the image that there may be an infection, but the only way to tell is to open you up and take cultures."

My face prickled as the blood drained out. I felt Dad's hand on my back. "It's okay," I said to him in my best tough-guy voice, but I was bawling inside. I couldn't believe what I had just heard.

Dr. C told us to head to the hospital first thing in the morning the next day. "We will perform surgery immediately."

Was this actually happening or was it a nightmare? If there was no bone there, that meant I might need yet another surgery to put in a prosthetic. If there was an infection, I would need a PIC line so they could administer IV antibiotics, and I might need additional treatments.

I had been so excited about enjoying my house with my friends that summer and living a normal life. My whole world had just come crashing down again. I was a complete wreck.

(ERICA)

THE ENTIRE FAMILY was at my parents' house celebrating Mother's Day. We were having fun. My cousin, Luke, and I were outside playing catch, which was somewhat of a ritual for us during family parties. I always looked forward to that because it was our chance to catch up and enjoy each other's company.

Joe came outside. I remember noticing the sun reflecting off his head. The shape of his head was not right. I felt an emptiness in my stomach. I didn't know what to do, but telling Joe was not an option.

Back in the house, I pulled my parents aside and told them what I had seen. I didn't want to scare them, but I was worried. They sneaked looks without telling Joe, and we all agreed that something definitely was off. We convinced ourselves that maybe the bone was reshaping itself, but looking back now, that didn't even make sense. It was just that none of us wanted to think about something being wrong.

Therefore, when Joe called to say he felt "off," I was certain that the doctor would say that he needed to go back into the hospital. And that's what happened. Joe needed another surgery.

We were on a never-ending rollercoaster ride! What the hell had Joe done to deserve all this? I thought about the hospital and seeing him with wires attached. I thought about him being in that stupid bed with nurses around. I knew I had to mentally prepare myself for it, but I couldn't do it. I was a wreck. I hid it from everyone. I vented to my friends and cried my eyes out. But to my brother, I just said that this was going to be a piece of cake. Nobody in this world could have made me feel better. Nobody in this world could have helped me understand why this was happening. Jesus himself could have come down and had a conversation with me, and it still wouldn't have justified or explained why Joe had to be in pain.

HERE WE GO AGAIN...
(JOE AND ERICA)

(JOE)

IT WAS NOT quite dawn on May 29, 2014. I was exhausted and petrified and had a bad headache. I couldn't take the headaches anymore, and I was terrified about what might happen during surgery.

I had started to fall asleep when medical personnel came in and took me to go through the typical pre-surgery procedures, which were way too familiar. When they asked me to do a test, I continued through the rest of the process without them having to tell me what to do next. I was nervous inside, but mostly, I was pissed off. Why had this happened to me? I was watching as my life slowly dragged on, hindered by speed bumps whenever I started to accelerate.

My parents and my sister were with me.

"Joe, are you okay?" Erica asked. "Are you nervous at all?"

I smiled and said, "Are you?"

She rolled her eyes. "Be honest with me."

I reassured them all. "I got this. Listen, I've been through worse. They'll take out the bone and test it for infections, and I'll be on my way." Honestly, it had become almost routine. "I can handle this. No problem."

We waited for hours. An emergency had come in that took priority. Finally, it was my turn.

Dr. C asked us if we had any questions before my surgery.

"Hey, when you open me up, none of those screws is going to fall into my brain, right?" I grinned.

"No, you're going to be okay. Don't worry."

I felt reassured; I really didn't want random screws in my brain.

As I was rolled away, I said, "I love you guys. I got this, I promise!" while holding my fist up in the air.

Then, five…four…three…two…one, and I was sound asleep.

"Give me medicine—now!" was the next thing I said—or rather, screamed.

I opened my eyes. I was still in the operating room. My surgery must have just finished. I was in excruciating pain. My head felt like it had been split wide open. It was ridiculously painful. I was cursing at everyone, which is not like me at all, but I couldn't help it. Instantly, I was given IV pain meds and icy coolness ran through my veins. I can see why some people get addicted. My pain and everything going on around me seemed far away, and I was glad. It was what I needed.

As I lay there, Dr. Baez, my infectious diseases doctor, came in and introduced himself. He gave me great news. They did a wash-out to clear away all bone particles and any potential infection. What was left of the bone had been about the size of a quarter and wafer-thin.

It was hard for me to believe that I had been walking around for who knows how long with virtually no bone on the right side of my head. What if I had gotten hit in the head while playing kickball? I could have lost my life!

I woke up groggy the next morning in what had become a familiar place. Dr. Baez arrived with results of the culture. "Okay, so we didn't see anything growing from the cultures last night, but as of this morning, we are starting to see the presence of a slow-growing staph infection. We will have a team come in to administer a PIC line."

Just what I was afraid of was happening. I was going to have a PIC line put in, and I would have to administer IV antibiotics for four to six weeks. Great, just great. And not only the PIC line and antibiotics, but I'd need to have a prosthetic skull to replace my bone.

Getting the PIC line put in was interesting. They covered everything in the room with plastic and put a sheet over me. It reminded me of TV shows where the bad guys set up everything carefully to kill someone and hide the evidence. I had to look away from where they would put the needle so I didn't breathe on the site. They put a tube in my right arm that went into a blood source that would lead directly into my heart and would dangle from my arm for up to six weeks.

It would be a rough time with a puppy at home and a life to live. How was I going to manage a tube that I had to keep ridiculously clean at all times? The whole situation was still hard for me to see as real. It could have been worse, though, I guessed.

My heart sank when hospital personnel came in to fit me for a new helmet: two summers in a row wearing a helmet. Did God not know how hot it was in that thing during the summer?

"Be positive, Joe," I told myself whenever I noticed I had drifted into negative thoughts. I wanted normalcy in my life, and I would continue moving forward.

A few days later, I was discharged from the hospital and sent home. I realized I had regressed despite all of the progress I made. My walking wasn't nearly as good at it had been, and my vision seemed much worse. Maybe the wash-out of my brain had made it swell a bit.

What else could I do but continue to follow the process? I didn't know what would happen; all I knew was that I wanted out of the helmet and wanted my normal life back.

A nurse came by once a week to check on my line and educate us on how to administer IV antibiotics, a chore that had turned my family into a bunch of nurses, as they had to do it several times a day. The antibiotics came in what looked like little plastic grenades filled with fluid. The connector at the end of the tube had to be cleaned with alcohol, and whoever administered the IV had to wear gloves to attach it to the PIC line. Then I had to sit there for 90 minutes or so a few times a day. Once a week, I went to Dr. Baez for a checkup. All I wanted to hear was that everything was fine and it was time to get measured for the prosthetic.

I had to be patient. My parents had raised me to work hard and never slack off. They told us nothing is given to you in life; instead, you have to work for it. I wanted to continue making money and supporting my team at work. I didn't want to let anyone down. I spent every weekday working from home to ensure that I was still a team player, and I hoped it wouldn't go unnoticed. I was in pain and deeply fatigued. I thought I probably should have gotten cleared by my rehab doctors before jumping right back into my life, but I didn't care. I had to continue to fight.

A couple of weeks later, my dad and I were together when we got awesome news. I had an appointment for an MRI, which would be used to take measurements for building my prosthetic. After that, Dr. Baez coordinated with Dr. C to determine when it was safe to put in the prosthetic and schedule my surgery. It had been a long, tiring journey.

I couldn't play with Bosco because I was nervous that he might touch the line. Once again, my family had been of huge help. They helped me walk him and play with him. My family members are my best friends, my supporters, and, well, they became a group of nurses. It was incredible how resilient we became as a family unit.

I enjoyed talking to Dr. Baez at my appointments. He was refreshingly down to earth and honest. He always focused on the positive and encouraged me to keep doing the same. I was extremely lucky that I'd been under the care of amazing doctors during my journey.

"Dr. Baez, when do you think I'll get my PIC line out?"

"Let me check how long it's been." He left to look up my chart and came back to examine the site where the PIC line went into my skin. He took the bandage off. "You're good. Let's get this PIC line out of you."

I was surprised. He held gauze over the area and did a little dance. I asked him if it would hurt when he pulled out the PIC line.

Why was he smiling? He held up his other hand and said, "You mean when *this* comes out?" He had already done it.

It felt weird not to have a tube in my arm. I was very happy!

I decided I would continue to work, but from home, until I knew the date of the surgery. A few days went by, and then my phone rang. My surgery would take place on July 30, 2014. That was only a week away. The end was in sight.

The night before, I was pumped. I was used to the whole night-before-surgery routine. I couldn't wait to be put back together again. I didn't want to feel nervous or anxious that time, but of course, I was, a little bit.

Just as I was about to be put under for surgery, I said, "Listen, this is the end of this ordeal. Once this is done, I'm good. I'm ready to close the final chapter of this journey."

Those were my last words to my family before being put under.

When my eyes opened, I was once again in terrific pain. They administered pain medication to ease me, and I saw my family. "It's over," I said to each one of them. Humpty Dumpty had been put back together again. In a couple of weeks, my staples would be removed and I'd be good as new. I couldn't wait!

(ERICA)

EVERYTHING WAS UP and down. First there was no infection; then there was; and then doctors were unsure. I didn't want to expect the best just to be let down. In the coffee shop at the hospital, I made the decision to just be strong. There was no other option. I couldn't even cry anymore. I felt let down. Just as life was finally back to whatever normalcy was left, and then this happened. With an infection, I knew we would have to be extremely careful.

After Joe's surgery, the surgeon came into the waiting room to explain what was going on. The only thing that stood out was that he'd had another patient a few years back that had gone through a number of infections before her nightmare was over.

All I could do was put my head in my hands and stop listening. I didn't see how I could watch my brother go through that. Finally, I cut the doctor off: "What do we need to do to make sure her nightmare doesn't happen to Joe?"

They would put a PIC line into Joe's arm that would go straight to his heart, and we would have to infuse him with several antibiotics over the next couple of months. I was surprised to hear that we would be doing that instead of a full-time nurse.

"Keep Joe in a place that is very clean, with clean sheets and clean towels. You will have to be extremely careful. Everyone will have to step up to the plate."

When the nurse came to explain what we would have to do with the antibiotics, I wrote everything down in detail and asked her to check it. Nobody would be able to make a mistake if I provided written directions.

At home, we had a routine. We determined that nothing bad was going to happen to my brother. Mom bought new sheets and towels that she bleached every day, and we were meticulous about the infusions.

Joe was back in a helmet and uncomfortable sleeping on one side. I hated that horrible helmet! I had thought that stupid thing was gone forever. It was like seeing my mortal enemy again after thinking he was gone for good.

Joe was a trouper, and so were my family. We took turns taking care of Bosco and infusing Joe. There wasn't one complaint. There was not one day when we worried that someone wouldn't be there to help him. We had to step up to the plate, and we did just that. Joe was alive, and he was going to stay that way!

SUMMER OF 2014
(JOE AND ERICA)

(JOE)

AFTER MY STAPLES were removed, I needed to make up for lost time. I spent time down the shore recovering with my family and going for long walks every day. I did my best to rehab on my own as much as possible.

All that had happened over the last several months had really scared me. Everything I did made me nervous. I didn't ever want the infection to return. I knew the staph infection was gone, but staph infections are tricky because they can so easily come back. I constantly took my temperature. Every time I had a headache, I got nervous that maybe my infection was coming back. It was no way to live. I was constantly on edge. Every day, I asked my parents if they saw anything that looked abnormal. It was taking a toll on me. I couldn't worry about this all the time. I decided that I needed to change my thinking. Gradually, I began to relax. I kept telling myself that there was nothing to worry about until there was something to worry about. I needed to be proactive and positive.

My dad and I talked about options for medical devices that had the potential give me a larger range of vision. I had come to terms with the impairment of my vision, and I wanted to try something innovative. Dad found some prism stickers that you stick on the lenses of a pair of glasses. They were a temporary solution so we could find out if I could get used to them. I figured, why not? The company mailed us the stickers, and I was back in business.

The waiting game continued. Things were looking up for me, and I couldn't wait to see what would happen next in my life. I had a feeling that from there on out, all good things were to come. No more detours in my life of positivity.

(ERICA)

I WORRIED THAT Joe might be upset about not being as independent as he used to be. During his hospital stay and his recovery, he was used to being surrounded by many people every day. We were still taking turns driving Joe to work and picking him up, but he needed his independence, and he needed it quickly. I could sense that he felt down sometimes, and it bothered me that I couldn't fix it for him. I had always helped him get through hard times until eventually things got better. But this situation was different. I couldn't fix his vision, and that was what was keeping him from being free to do as he pleased.

Dad never gave up on looking for a solution. Together, he and Joe looked up many different programs and devices that might help Joe regain his independence, and I was happy to hear that they had found some prism stickers to try. I just wanted something, anything, to work. Joe needed to be on the move again for the sake of his self-esteem. Seeing him upset about his situation killed me inside. I felt a sense of guilt that this was happening to him and I couldn't do anything to make it better. His physical pain became my mental and emotional pain.

I realized that all our lives might change forever. If he couldn't drive, I would have to move closer to him. Of course I didn't mind that, but I had to stay close to his situation so I would know exactly how I needed to help him. I would dedicate my life to making sure he was as independent as he could be. Joe and I had always shared our dreams, and I was determined not to let this situation kill even one of them. I would do what I had to do to help him.

I thank God for my family every day. We are the greatest team in the world. Each of us had played a huge role in Joe's recovery. We had spotted each other. When one of us needed some downtime, another stepped up to the plate. Some families crumble when confronted with situations that are difficult. Not us. We were an even stronger unit than we had been because of the situation.

BACK TO REHAB
(JOE AND ERICA)

(JOE)

BY THE MIDDLE of August 2014, I had reached the point in my recovery where I was no longer going to worry and make myself sick over whether I might catch another bad break. I wanted to turn up the intensity. I wanted to run, jump, and sprint. I knew I could do it if I worked hard enough. It would take time and tremendous effort, but I was capable of doing it. So I went back to Kessler to do more outpatient physical therapy.

Physical therapy was not like it was the first time. Some days, it felt like basic training. They started with an assessment exam.

I tried skipping, and I didn't get very far. I tried running down the hall, but I was slow. I tried jumping over small hurdles, but I knocked them over. It was rough. I may have been a year out, but I was determined that my recovery wouldn't end with the condition I was in. At home, I practiced standing on my toes and walking on the balls of my feet. I took longer walks with Bosco. I walked, jogged, and jumped as best I could. I wasn't very good at it, but I knew I would be eventually.

After a few sessions, I knew how hard I needed to push myself, and Tyler, my physical therapist, was happy to push me to the limits.

We jogged in the parking lot. I walked up and down the stairs holding weights, but that wasn't enough, so I held awkward cylinder weights that made it more difficult. I worked on a leg-press machine. I stretched. I felt like I was in boot camp.

I did these sessions for a few months twice a week. In November, they did another assessment. I ran down the hall in a much faster time, and I could skip. My jumping had improved to the point that I was doing an exercise I hadn't been able to do when I first tried. Incredibly, I was attaining all the goals I had set for myself physically.

Mom was waiting for me outside the gym after the assessment. I jumped, ran, and skipped out of the waiting area.

"I told you I got this!"

I had officially graduated from outpatient physical therapy. It was a great day! I would be able to return to work in December of 2014. This time, I was ready.

(ERICA)

I WAS THRILLED to see that Joe didn't stop where he was. He went back to rehab determined to work hard to make as much of a recovery as he could. I'd see him running and doing exercises that I hadn't thought even I could do! For one exercise, he sat on a chair with wheels and zipped right by me using just his legs. He was fast! I heard one woman whispering to her husband, "Why is he even at Kessler? He looks absolutely fine." That was a great conversation to overhear! My brother, the guy who had been so down and negative, was now positive and determined to be the best version of himself. I loved the new and improved Joe!

I watched him as he worked out at Kessler on some days. Sometimes, I saw Joe looking at me. He impressed himself, but I really think he wanted to see my reaction. Of course, I was always happy and proud of progress. He was getting so strong that I felt that one day this situation would be nothing but a memory. Joe would make such a wonderful recovery that his life would be even better because this thing had happened to him.

NEVER SAY NEVER
(JOE AND ERICA)

(JOE)

BY THE MIDDLE of November, I'd been practicing with the stick-on prisms for my glasses for a week or so and getting used them. To make sure I had them on correctly, Dad and I took a trip into New York City to see Dr. Bryan, an eye doctor at Glasses On First. Dr. Bryan Wolynski knew about the prisms and was eager to work with me to ensure I had the optimal lenses and that the prisms were affixed correctly. Dr. Bryan and I connected well. He asked me to tell him my story. I mentioned my passion for helping people. "I know I'm going to make a difference someday. I will give back and do something good with all that has happened to me," I said.

Dr. Bryan shared with me the cool things he does to help the community and those in need. After going through what I had, I had great respect for him. We instantly became friends. I left with new lenses with my stick-on prisms to try for a couple of weeks. They worked for me, and I returned to get the permanent prisms etched into the glass. These give me an even wider range of vision than the stickers.

I didn't know how much improvement to expect. When Dr. Bryan handed me the new pair and I tried them on, I was astounded at how much more I could see. My vision was even better than I had thought it would be. Everything looked much clearer through the etched prisms than it had with the stickers. I was ready to practice with them as much as possible, ready to do my exercises with them. In the car that first day, my dad asked me how they were. "I can see that car coming from the left." I said. I filled up with tears of happiness, and so did my dad.

On December 1st, 2014, I returned to work, wearing my prisms. A week or so later, I made a big decision: I made an appointment at Kessler for the Driver Rehabilitation program. I would be required to pass a series of tests at Kessler to determine if I was capable to drive safely. My appointment was for just before Christmas. I went into overdrive. I practiced my eye exercises every day, and every day I became more comfortable.

That was the biggest moment of my life. I was facing a test that had the potential to give me back my independence. The worst depression and slump I'd ever had hit me after I went to see the neuro-ophthalmologist, who stripped me of any hope. I wanted to prove Dr. Insensitive wrong so badly.

The series of tests were to evaluate my vision, reflexes, timing, and understanding of road rules. Last was the road test. I got in the car and drove around for an hour with the instructor. When we pulled back up to Kessler, I didn't know what the instructor was going to say. I had driven well. I've always been a cautious and defensive driver, and I was especially cautious after what I'd been through.

"Park over there so we can talk," my instructor said.

My heart was racing in anticipation as to what was to follow. After I had parked, he said, "Listen, you've been through a lot. You did a really good job driving. You exercised extreme caution. I felt safer in the car with you than I do with some people who have never been through anything like you have. Congratulations, Joe. You can go buy yourself that car that you wanted."

I had done it. I had proved that doctor wrong. I had tackled my biggest goal and won.

Later, I met Dad in the cafeteria. I said, "I just want to hurry and get coffee and get out of here," with my sad face on.

"What happened? What's wrong?" he said, concerned.

"I want to get to the car dealer before the traffic gets heavy." I grinned.

We hugged, both of us in tears.

"I did it. I told you I was going to do it!" I said proudly.

I couldn't wait to tell Erica and Mom. I had defied all the odds. We went to the car dealer and I signed the paperwork for my car.

It was December 24, 2014. God definitely was watching over me during my journey. That Christmas was the best Christmas of my life. God is good!

(ERICA)

THE DAY MY brother bought his new car was the best moment of the entire ordeal. I really hadn't been convinced that Joe would drive again; clearly, I was wrong. I canceled my plans that afternoon. When I pulled up at his house, I saw his new car. It looked awesome! I knew how happy he must be.

He showed me every feature the car had, and it took longer than the tour he had given me when he moved into his new house. I wanted to treat him to a steak dinner that night to celebrate. I climbed into his car for the first time in ages.

The second I sat down, I felt nervous and emotional all at the same time. We'd taken so many car rides together in the past, blasting the music and singing along to stupid songs. That time was a bit different. We had the music low. Joe didn't move that car until he was positive that it was safe. I was proud of him.

"Sit in the back seat," he said, once we had parked at the restaurant. Then, he hit a button. The headrests fell and smacked me in the back of the head. He had been waiting for that moment for the entire ride. Joe was back in business!

I was impressed with his driving and how careful he was. Of course I had been worried, but actually getting into the car with him had eased many of my fears. After a few more rides, I knew he would be able to get to work safely. Practice would make perfect. Just knowing that his independence was possible felt great. The huge weight I'd carried from the beginning of this was lifted.

Seeing Joe happy was like the best drug for my parents and me. His smile was contagious, and we would do anything to see it.

LIFE GOES ON (JOE AND ERICA)

(JOE)

IT'S NOW 2016. My life continues to take shape after nearly losing it. Quite often, I catch myself looking back on what I've been through. It seems surreal.

Before June 9, 2013, I'd never had any surgeries. I wish I had been eased into it with something minor, but that's okay. I now know that I can handle anything that is thrown my way. I learn more about the new me every day. Every experience helps me understand my new norm. I'd be lying if I said everything is easy, because that is the furthest thing from the truth. Actually, the hardest part about my recovery is getting to know who this new version of me is.

Almost every day, I catch myself thinking about doing something I did before my brain bleed. Then I realize that it might be a struggle now. For example, at times I attempt to run up the stairs as I used to, and I'm quickly hit with the reality that my left leg just doesn't move the way it used to. Situations like this, since they occur on a daily basis, killed me emotionally for a long time. They are constant reminders of what once was and now isn't. I knew I couldn't go on being down every time I thought of something I once loved to do and now cannot. That is not who I was or am, and not who I will be. I can't box or play in a pickup game of basketball anymore, but what I can do is punch a bag or hit mitts, shoot a basketball with friends, watch sports on TV, and go to meet athletes and further build my autographed memorabilia collection. I have learned to focus on what I still have and not on what I lost.

I still *do not* have full sensation on my left side, I get headaches on a daily basis, and I suffer from severe fatigue. These changes are all fine, though, because I *do have* some sensation on my left, I *can* take medicine for my headaches, *I can* open my eyes every morning, and last, I'm *alive*. I do tend to look at my life as before and after the rupture, but I do it in a positive way. I was happy with the person I was before, but I am more pleased with who I have become. I'm excited to share my message with the world and to use my story for the good of others. I am giving back. I regularly go back to Overlook and Kessler to inspire and give hope to those going through similar situations.

I have said it before and I will continue to say it for the rest of my life:

Anything really is possible if you want it badly enough.

(ERICA)

DURING JOE'S ORDEAL, going to work every day was a great distraction. I love what I do for a living, so being around so many great people truly helped. My students needed me, and, to be honest, I needed them. I was responsible for things that I couldn't let fall through the cracks. Students needed my help through all of the emotional middle school stressors. Plus, I knew that keeping busy was key.

That's not to say that I didn't feel overwhelmed at times. There were moments when I had to sit down in my office with the door shut just to catch my breath. At times, I was very emotional. I'd sit at my desk and stare at my cell phone. I felt like I was waiting for someone to call with some kind of bad news. My anxiety sometimes got the better of me. I was at the edge of my seat waiting for my world to crash down on me. I realized that this was horrible and irrational, but I had zero control over how I felt.

A few close coworkers were rock stars for me. They were there for me through it all. They looked after me and made sure that I was not getting overwhelmed. Yes, work was my escape, but it was also time spent with amazing people who truly cared. They knew when I was upset, and there was no way they were going to let me deal with this on my own. I know how lucky I am to have a second family that I get to call coworkers.

I felt like I was missing so much while I was at work. I was used to seeing Joe every day, and I was sad not to have that anymore. However, I realized that it meant that Joe was independent again, and living his life. And there is nothing in this world that I want more.

FINAL WORDS
(ERICA AND JOE)

(ERICA)

I'M A DAUGHTER, a counselor, a friend, and a sister. I take these four roles seriously. Through this experience, I learned something about myself in each of these roles.

As a daughter, I learned that I have the best parents in the world. In all of the time that my brother was going through hell, they never complained once. My parents were there for him, for me, and for each other.

I'd go to sleep before my father and wake up to find that he was gone. He spent every waking moment with my brother, and for that, I will never in my life question his value or his unconditional love for his children. When my brother and I were growing up, Dad sometimes mentioned that he wanted to be the kind of father to my brother and me that his father was to him. Sometimes, I wondered whether he felt that he could fill his father's shoes. I can only hope that Dad now realizes that, in my eyes, he surpasses any expectations that Joe and I ever had. He has filled his father's shoes and then some.

Mom kept to herself at first. She repressed her feelings, and that worried me. Now I realize that she turned to God throughout the experience. Without her love and guidance, I probably would have sworn off my faith completely. I was angry. I couldn't understand why this had happened to Joe. There were times when I mentioned that God didn't protect him. I watched my mom pray every day, without fail. Eventually, I realized that she had depended upon her faith to get her through. She was not angry with God. She was thankful that God had kept my brother alive and helped him throughout his recovery. I've always looked up to my mom, but to say that she is my best friend and role model would be an understatement. I am proud to be her daughter, and every single day of my life, I work my hardest to be the kind of person who makes her proud.

My aunt also showed great strength. I saw how much she took care of my parents. She was my mom's rock and never left her side. She took care of things without being asked. Her relationship with my mom is very close, similar to the relationship Joe and I have. She is the one who experienced the most horrific day of my life with me. Only we know how scary it was to see Joe in that horrible state. She didn't let me go there alone, and for that, I will be forever grateful. I am lucky enough to have yet another family member who has been like a parent to me.

My entire family impressed me. Each of them took care of my parents, my brother, and me, anticipating what we would need. They spent countless hours and days with us in the hospital and the rehab hospital. My family is my whole heart. They will always be my reason for breathing. I would do anything for any of them.

As a counselor, I learned just how therapeutic my students could be. Without even knowing it, they helped me to survive. No people are more genuine, vulnerable, and kind than children. They were a good outlet and resource for me. When helping them and listening to some of their thoughts regarding their concerns, I learned more about life and about me. I genuinely love what I do for a living, and now I realize how much I value the students I've worked with.

Since I work in a small town, word got around quickly that my brother was in the hospital. Some parents of my students called to check in on me. They went out of their way to make sure I was okay. The phone calls, emails, and conversations that I had with these families helped me get through the worst time of my life. I appreciate these people so much, and they will always hold a special place in my heart.

As a friend, I learned that there are people who are in our lives for a reason. As I've mentioned throughout my portions of this book, I have always been extremely appreciative of the people who were there for me. I believe I had some close friends who were meant to be in my life as a support system just for this one experience alone. And that's okay, because that's how life works. Maybe that was why they were with me. Some aren't around anymore, but I'll always wish them the best because they distracted me when I couldn't deal with things on my own. My faith has allowed me to believe that God works in mysterious ways. He takes people out of your life sometimes because they're not good for you in the long run. I don't question God's intentions anymore. I go with the flow, and my faith allows me to be okay with that!

On the other end, there are those lifetime friends whose support I will never forget: friends who sat with me in the hospital and let me cry; friends who took time during their busiest moments to listen to me when I called from the emergency room; friends who took the time to visit. I also had friends who arranged for celebrities to call and wish my brother well. I had friends and coworkers who asked about my brother, and then asked about me. And although I didn't ever want the focus to be on my feelings, they wouldn't allow me to get away with that. They were my strength when I didn't have any left. They will forever be my best friends, and I will always appreciate them more than I can express.

And now for one of my most important roles: I am a sister. And not just any sister. I am a sister to Joseph Anthony Slota III, a superhero, a walking miracle, and the best brother a girl could ask for. My brother and I were raised to be close—we were raised right! We have always been there for each other. It's been about picking each other up when we need it. Joe's experience scared me more than anything I've ever experienced. Losing my brother was something I had never considered. While I waited in the waiting room of the ER on that very first night, I thought about what it would be like to not have him. I couldn't handle the thought, even though I knew there was a strong chance that it could be my reality.

My brother defied all odds. Despite some of Joe's physical deficits, he is a better person today than he was three years ago. His compassion, love, and values are unconditional and endless. I loved him very much before this happened to him, but I don't think I realized how strong both of us could be when going through hell. We did it. We did it together. He is my only brother, and I am his only sister. We are the only people who could ever fill those shoes. When Joe can't see something to his left, I tell him what's there. When I feel down, he picks me up. We will spend the rest of our lives making up for the other's deficits when needed, which, in the end, depletes those deficits! My brother is my hero.

Throughout this experience, we met many people. Race, religion, gender, sexual orientation, and so forth meant absolutely nothing to any of us. People from all walks of life worked hard to help my brother progress. Ignorant, worldly attitudes didn't exist in any of those interactions. We were all people with a common goal. This open-minded attitude should exist throughout our world. People should work together to make our world a more positive place. People of all kinds saved my brother. Who knows what could happen in our society if everyone had that same goal?

An experience like ours can throw a wrench in every plan you ever had. So live each day to its fullest, and be good to the people around you. Take that extra time to build on your core values. Love what you do and the people you surround yourself with. Most important, love yourself with all your heart, because that's truly the only way to develop enough strength to see yourself through the hard experiences in life.

May life be kind to each of you who read this book. And if it is unkind at some point, I hope our words will inspire you. Thank you for reading.

(JOE)

MY NAME IS Joseph Anthony Slota III, and I am walking proof that *anything is possible if you want it badly enough.*

Before June 9, 2013, I was just your average guy. I'm no longer that average guy. With the support of family and friends, I was able to keep positive, determined, and resilient and achieve my goals throughout my recovery. Help me to achieve my greatest lifelong goal of using my story for the good of others. I was dealt a bad hand, but it happened for a reason, and I accept that. It took me a while to come to terms with the new me, but here I am with a smile on my face and feeling more determined than ever. Help me spread my message. *Anything is possible if you want it badly enough.*

If the story of my journey helps at least one person, then I am happy this happened to me. No one deserves to suffer, especially alone. Every recovery has its ups and downs, but it's how you choose to overcome the downs that will make you successful. I will not consider myself recovered until I know that I am able to help others overcome a difficult situation. Help me to recover. Think positively. Be resilient. Don't give up. Smile. Laugh. Fight. Love. *Anything is possible.*

Thank you for helping me to recover! God bless!

Joseph Anthony Slota III

A GUIDE TO WEATHER THE STORM (JOE AND ERICA)

(JOE)

1. Set small, achievable goals.
2. Remain positive.
3. Keep a sense of humor. Laughter really is the best medicine.
4. Believe in yourself.
5. Use any negativity as motivation to succeed.
6. Everyone is entitled to have a bad day.
7. Don't resist resting.
8. Celebrate the small accomplishments.
9. Don't bottle up your feelings. There's no shame in talking to someone.
10. Surround yourself with positive people who make you feel good about your progress.
11. Keep fighting, because "no" is never an answer to whether or not you can achieve your goals.

12. Never stop looking for answers. You'll only be cheating yourself if you do.

13. You can only control so much. Focus on every situation and think about what you can control and work at that.

14. Understand that the old you is not gone. The old you is very much alive in the new version of you. Embrace it and come to terms with it over time.

15. Truly believe in your heart of hearts that anything is possible if you want it badly enough.

(ERICA)

1. Breathe.

2. Listen to *everything*.

3. Lean on others.

4. Take care of yourself.

5. Communicate.

6. Try to keep your faith.

7. Know your limitations.

8. Rest.

9. Prepare for the worst, but hope for the best.

10. Ask questions.

11. Never give up.

12. Love with your whole heart.

ABOUT THE AUTHORS

Joseph Anthony Slota III is a ruptured brain AVM survivor with an ambitious goal to dedicate his life and his story to helping others to be resilient. He resides in New Jersey, where he has lived his entire life. At twenty-six years old, his brain AVM ruptured, resulting in a fight for his life. While working through his rehabilitation, Joe identified his passion and purpose in life, which is to help others overcome challenging life obstacles. Before the rupture, he had a successful career in professional services and technology companies. After his rupture, he set out on a journey to use his story for the good of others while continuing his career.

Erica Slota has her master's degree in counseling and is a middle school counselor. She is passionate about her work and looks forward to learning something new from her students every day. Erica enjoys spending time with friends and family, traveling to new places, and helping others. She has great pride in and respect for her brother, who showed extreme resilience throughout his recovery.

JosephAnthonySlota.com

Made in the USA
San Bernardino, CA
16 July 2019